D1810815

Essentials of Sports Nutrition

Essentials of Sports Nutrition

Tobias Fry

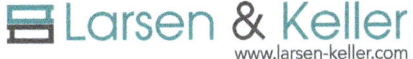
Larsen & Keller
www.larsen-keller.com

Essentials of Sports Nutrition
Tobias Fry
ISBN: 978-1-64172-697-9 (Hardback)

© 2021 Larsen & Keller

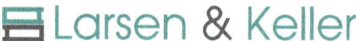 Larsen & Keller

Published by Larsen and Keller Education,
5 Penn Plaza,
19th Floor,
New York, NY 10001, USA

Cataloging-in-Publication Data

Essentials of sports nutrition / Tobias Fry.
    p. cm.
Includes bibliographical references and index.
ISBN 978-1-64172-697-9
1. Athletes--Nutrition. 2. Athletes--Health and hygiene. 3. Exercise--Physiological aspects.
4. Sports--Physiological aspects. 5. Physical fitness--Nutritional aspects. I. Fry, Tobias.
TX361.A8 E87 2021
613.202 479 6--dc23

This book contains information obtained from authentic and highly regarded sources. All chapters are published with permission under the Creative Commons Attribution Share Alike License or equivalent. A wide variety of references are listed. Permissions and sources are indicated; for detailed attributions, please refer to the permissions page. Reasonable efforts have been made to publish reliable data and information, but the authors, editors and publisher cannot assume any responsibility for the validity of all materials or the consequences of their use.

Trademark Notice: All trademarks used herein are the property of their respective owners. The use of any trademark in this text does not vest in the author or publisher any trademark ownership rights in such trademarks, nor does the use of such trademarks imply any affiliation with or endorsement of this book by such owners.

For more information regarding Larsen and Keller Education and its products, please visit the publisher's website www.larsen-keller.com

Table of Contents

Preface

The purpose of this book is to help students understand the fundamental concepts of this discipline. It is designed to motivate students to learn and prosper. I am grateful for the support of my colleagues. I would also like to acknowledge the encouragement of my family.

Sports nutrition includes the study of diet and nutrition related to sports to improve the athletic performance. It is primarily required in endurance sports such as cycling, running and swimming, and in strength sports like bodybuilding and weightlifting. Sports nutrition focuses on the food quantity that is consumed by an athlete. It also looks after the consumption of organic substances such as carbohydrates, fats and proteins as well as the consumption of nutrients including minerals, vitamins and supplements. The dietary ingredients such as amino acids and herbs in the form of pills, capsules and liquid are included as the dietary supplements. There are various factors that influence the nutritional requirements. They include the type of activity, weight, gender, body mass index, height, and the workout stage. This book explores all the important aspects of sports nutrition in the present day scenario. The topics covered herein deal with the core subjects of sports nutrition. Those in search of information to further their knowledge will be greatly assisted by this book.

A foreword for all the chapters is provided below:

Chapter – Introduction

Sports nutrition deals with the study of implementing appropriate diet and nutrition to improve the athletic performance of a sportsperson. It studies the energy-yielding nutrients, energy balance, and quantity of fluids and ideal food taken by an athlete. The topics elaborated in this chapter will help in gaining a better perspective about sports nutrition.

Chapter – Exercise and Nutrition

Exercise and nutrition enhance and maintain the physical fitness and overall health of athletes. It includes the concepts of anti-oxidants, hydration, pre and post-exercise nutrition, etc. This chapter has been carefully written to provide an easy understanding of these concepts under exercise and nutrition.

Chapter – Sports Drinks, Foods and Supplements

Sports drinks are used to prevent dehydration and maintain the body's balance of fluids at an optimum level. Sports food, protein bars, energy gels, whey protein, soy protein, etc. are used by athletes for increasing the efficiency in their performance. This chapter discusses these sports drinks, foods and supplements in detail.

Chapter – Adverse Effects of Supplements

Supplements affect the health of the athletes adversely. It can cause bloating, muscle cramps, nausea, stroke, heart diseases, liver damage, high cholesterol, high blood pressure, infertility, etc. This chapter closely examines these adverse effects of supplements to provide an extensive understanding of the subject.

Chapter – Weight Management for Athletes

Weight management is important for improving athletic performance and helps in preventing the development of serious chronic diseases. A few of its aspects include body mass index, calorie restriction, weight gain and loss strategies, etc. All these weight management strategies for athletes have been carefully analyzed in this chapter.

Chapter – Daily Meal Plans for Athletes

Different meal plans are necessary for various kinds of sports such as cricket, cycling, climbing, wrestling, bodybuilding, swimming, running, etc. This chapter sheds light on different meal plans for athletes associated with various sports to provide an in-depth understanding of the subject.

Tobias Fry

1

Introduction

Sports nutrition deals with the study of implementing appropriate diet and nutrition to improve the athletic performance of a sportsperson. It studies the energy-yielding nutrients, energy balance, and quantity of fluids and ideal food taken by an athlete. The topics elaborated in this chapter will help in gaining a better perspective about sports nutrition.

Nutrition

Nutrition is the combination of elements consumed by a person that nourishes the body, enabling it to sustain in an efficient manner all of its functions. Nutritionists seek to further understand by objective scientific method the nutritional needs of people to attain health and avoid disease and artfully try to work with people's varied lifestyles, cultural heritages, and tastes to enable those needs to be met through enjoyable eating patterns.

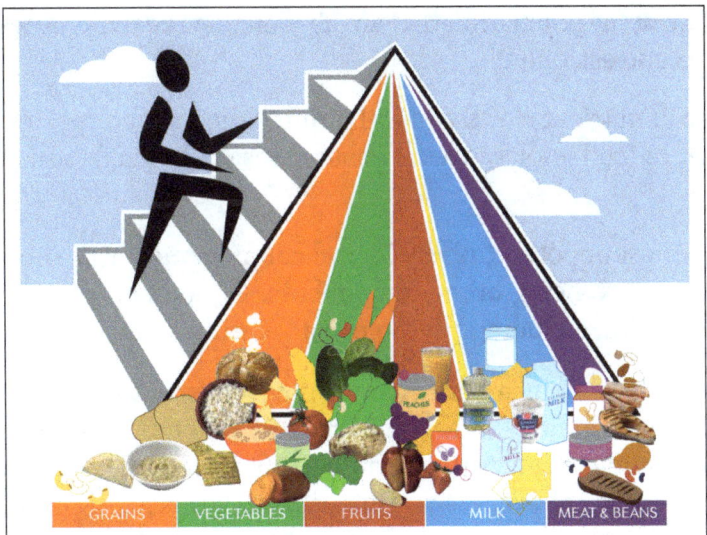

Food pyramid.

Deficiencies, excesses, and imbalances in diet can produce negative impacts on health, which may lead to diseases such as scurvy, obesity, or osteoporosis, as well as psychological and behavioral problems. Moreover, excessive ingestion of elements that have no apparent role in health, (e.g. lead, mercury, PCBs, dioxins), may incur toxic and potentially lethal effects, depending on the dose.

Although many organisms can survive on a limited variety of food sources, human nutrition is aided through the relationship with a vast array of plants and animals. To gain all the amino acids, fatty acids, carbohydrates, vitamins, and other nutriments necessary for good health, it is recommended that humans have a varied diet, which may include fish, seaweed, whole grains and legumes, nuts and seeds, vegetables and fruits, and so forth. Even microorganisms play a role in human nutrition, as a symbiotic relationship with bacteria in the gut aids digestion.

Internal aspects are also important, as digestion is aided by a good mood and hindered when under stress.

Nutrition relates to individual and social responsibility. On the one hand, personal discipline is required to have a good diet. On the other hand, people have a responsibility to care for society at large, such as aiding those without means for proper nutrition, overseeing the processing of foods that may be inexpensive but lack nutritional value, and investigating and educating on what constitutes a good dietary lifestyle.

The science of nutrition attempts to understand how and why specific dietary aspects influence health.

Nutritional knowledge is applied in four broad areas:

- Firstly, the general population, as world governments and individuals are concerned with the general health and productivity capacity of people.

- Secondly, people in emergencies—whether they be from natural disasters or conflict zones—supporting refugees to survive or those in hospitals who can not feed themselves.

- Thirdly, sections of the population that are challenging the boundaries of human limitation such as athletes and astronauts.

- Finally, the use of nutrients for those with limited dietary choices, to counter the impact of genes, allergies, or food intolerances to ensure these individuals still their nutritional needs fulfilled.

Nutrition is one of the most important physiological components for the body's good health, with fresh water, air, and exercise being other components. Of course, there are other contributing elements to a person's health, including psychological, spiritual, and social aspects.

Nutrition science seeks to explain metabolic and physiological responses of the body to diet. With advances in molecular biology, biochemistry, and genetics, nutrition science is additionally developing into the study of integrative metabolism, which seeks to connect diet and health through the lens of biochemical processes. Nutritionists are seeking to know which chemical components of food supply energy, regulate body processes, or promote the growth and repair of body tissue.

The RDA (recommended daily intake) relates to essential nutrients considered to be adequate to meet the nutritional needs of healthy people with moderate levels of activity. Although all persons have the need for the same nutrients, the amounts of the nutrients required by an individual are influenced by age, sex, body size, environment, level of activity, and nutritional status. The nutritional status of a person can be assessed by evaluation of dietary intake, anthropometric measurement, health assessment and laboratory tests.

The human body is made up of chemical compounds such as water, amino acids (proteins), fatty acids (lipids), nucleic acids (DNA/RNA), and carbohydrates (e.g. sugars and fiber). These compounds in turn consist of elements such as carbon, hydrogen, oxygen, nitrogen, and phosphorus, and may or may not contain minerals such as calcium, iron, or zinc. Minerals ubiquitously occur in the form of salts and electrolytes.

All of these chemical compounds and elements occur in various forms and combinations (e.g. hormones/vitamins, phospholipids, hydroxyapatite), both in the human body and in organisms (e.g. plants, animals) that humans eat. All of the essential elements must be present, and for some with certain genetic conditions where they lack a certain enzyme such that other nutrients are not manufactured by the body, these must be supplied in the diet as well. Adequate and properly proportioned nutrition gives a person more options in life, enabling them to have the resources they need to fulfill their daily activities.

In general, eating a variety of fresh, whole (unprocessed) plant foods has proven hormonally and metabolically favorable compared to eating a monotonous diet based on processed foods. In particular, consumption of whole plant foods slows digestion and provides higher amounts and a more favorable balance of essential and vital nutrients per unit of energy; resulting in better management of cell growth, maintenance, and mitosis (cell division) as well as regulation of blood glucose and appetite. A generally more regular eating pattern (e.g. eating medium-sized meals every 3 to 4 hours) has also proven more hormonally and metabolically favorable than infrequent, haphazard food intake.

Nutrition and Health

There are six main nutrients which the body needs to receive. These nutrients are proteins, fats, carbohydrates, vitamins, minerals, and water.

It is important to consume these six nutrients on a daily basis to build and maintain healthy body systems. What the body is able to absorb through the small intestine into the blood stream—and from there into individual cells—is influenced by many factors, especially the efficiency of the digestive system, which is why two people of similar build may eat the same food but will have different nutritional outcomes.

Ill health can be caused by an imbalance of nutrients, producing either an excess or deficiency, which in turn affects body functioning cumulatively. Moreover, because most nutrients are, in some way or another, involved in cell-to-cell signaling (e.g. as building blocks or part of hormone or signaling "cascades"), deficiency or excess of various nutrients affects hormonal function indirectly.

Thus, because they largely regulate the expression of genes, hormones represent a link between nutrition and how our genes are expressed, i.e. our phenotype. The strength and nature of this link are continually under investigation, but observations especially in recent years have demonstrated a pivotal role for nutrition in hormonal activity and function and, therefore, in health.

Essential and Non-essential Amino Acids

The body requires amino acids to produce new body protein (protein retention) and to replace damaged proteins (maintenance) that are lost in the urine.

Protein is the major functional and structural component of all the cells in the body. It is needed, for example, to form hormones, enzymes, antibodies for the immune system, blood transport molecules, and nucleic acids, as well as build the muscles, blood and its vessels, skin, hair, liver, and brain. If there are insufficient carbohydrates or oils in the diet, protein can be used as an inefficient form of heat and energy.

In animals, amino acid requirements are classified in terms of essential (an animal cannot produce them) and non-essential (the animal can produce them from other nitrogen containing compounds. Consuming a diet that contains adequate amounts of essential (but also non-essential) amino acids is particularly important for growing animals, who have a particularly high requirement.

Protein is provided in the diet by eating flesh foods (fish, eggs, chickens, and meat) and the combining of lentils or other legumes with brown rice, millet, or buckwheat; or legumes with nuts or seeds (hence the value of hommus as a economical effective protein source for many parts of the world). Inadequate protein in the diet can lead to kwashiorkor. If calories and protein are inadequate, protein-calorie malnutrition occurs.

Fatty Acids

Although most fatty acids can be manufacture by the body from dietary oils, carbohydrates and proteins, there are two essential fatty acids that need to be consumed. These two are linoleic acid and linolenic acid.

The RDA ("recommended daily allowance," or "recommended daily intake," RDI) for the essential fatty acids (EFA) is one to two percent of total energy intake. Persons at risk for EFA deficiency tend to be the same as those at risk for fat soluble vitamin deficiencies, especially vitamin E. Some signs are shared by the deficiencies. The most specific sign for linoleic acid deficiency is eczematous dermatitis. Premature infants, infants from poorly nourished mothers, and those suffering fat malabsorption syndromes tend to become deficient. As well, those who have the EFAs in the trans form rather than the cis would experience this. The body can only use the trans form as fuels and not as part of the essential functions.

The essential fatty acids are the starting point for the manufacture of prostaglandins, leukotrienes, prostcyclins, and thromboxanes. They alter the removal of low density lipoproteins and promote reduction of cholesterol. EPAs also are part of the structure of phospholipids in all cell membranes. Furthermore, EPAs are needed for neural function in the brain and eyes, and are needed for the synthesis of myelin.

Linolenic acid belongs to the family of omega-3 fatty acids (polyunsaturated fatty acids with a carbon-carbon double bond in the ω-3 position) and linoleic acid belongs to the family of omega-6 fatty acids (the first double bond in the carbon backbone occurs in the omega minus 6 position). In addition to sufficient intake of the essential fatty acids, an appropriate balance of omega-3 and omega-6 fatty acids has been discovered to be crucial for maintaining health. Both of these unique "omega" long-chain polyunsaturated fatty acids are substrates for a class of eicosanoids known as prostaglandins that function as hormones. The omega-3 eicosapentaenoic acid (EPA) (which can be made in the body from the omega-3 essential fatty acid alpha-linolenic acid (LNA), or taken in through marine food sources), serves as building block for series 3 prostaglandins (e.g. weakly-inflammation PGE3). The omega-6 dihomo-gamma-linolenic acid (DGLA) serves as building block for series 1 prostaglandins (e.g. anti-inflammatory PGE1), whereas arachidonic acid (AA) serves as building block for series 2 prostaglandins (e.g. pro-inflammatory PGE 2). Both DGLA and AA are made from the omega-6 linoleic acid (LA) in the body, or can be taken in directly through food. An appropriately balanced intake of omega-3 and omega-6 partly determines the relative production of different prostaglandins, which partly explains the importance of omega-3/omega-6 balance for cardiovascular health. In industrialized societies, people generally consume large amounts of processed vegetable oils that have reduced amounts of essential fatty acids along with an excessive amount of omega-6 relative to omega-3.

The rate of conversions of omega-6 DGLA to AA largely determines the production of the respective prostaglandins PGE1 and PGE2. Omega-3 EPA prevents AA from being released from membranes, thereby skewing prostaglandin balance away from pro-inflammatory PGE2 made from AA toward anti-inflammatory PGE1 made from DGLA. Moreover, the conversion (desaturation) of DGLA to AA is controlled by the enzyme delta-5-desaturase, which in turn is controlled by hormones such as insulin (up-regulation) and glucagon (down-regulation). Because different types and amounts of food eaten/absorbed affect insulin, glucagon, and other hormones to varying degrees, not only the amount of omega-3 versus omega-6 eaten but also the general composition of the diet therefore determine health implications in relation to essential fatty acids, inflammation (e.g. immune function) and mitosis (i.e. cell division).

Sugars

Glucose, the currency of energy for the body, is available from some fruit and vegetables directly, but also through the digestion and processing of other carbohydrates, fats, and proteins. The deficiency and excess consumption of sufficient energy components has serious repercussions for health.

Several lines of evidence indicate lifestyle-induced hyperinsulinemia (excess levels of circulating insulin in blood) and reduced insulin function (i.e. insulin resistance) as a decisive factor in many disease states. For example, hyperinsulinemia and insulin resistance are strongly linked to chronic inflammation, which in turn is strongly linked to a variety of adverse developments, such as arterial microinjuries and clot formation (i.e. heart disease) and exaggerated cell division (i.e. cancer). Hyperinsulinemia and insulin resistance (the so-called metabolic syndrome) are characterized by a combination of abdominal obesity, elevated blood sugar, elevated blood pressure, elevated blood triglycerides, and reduced HDL cholesterol. The negative impact of hyperinsulinemia on prostaglandin PGE1/PGE2 balance may be significant.

The state of obesity clearly contributes to insulin resistance, which in turn can cause type 2 diabetes. Virtually all obese and most type 2 diabetic individuals have marked insulin resistance. Although the association between overfatness and insulin resistance is clear, the exact (likely multifarious) causes of insulin resistance remain less clear. Importantly, it has been demonstrated that appropriate exercise, more regular food intake, and reducing glycemic load all can reverse insulin resistance in overfat individuals (and thereby lower blood sugar levels in those who have type 2 diabetes).

Obesity can unfavorably alter hormonal and metabolic status via resistance to the hormone leptin, and a vicious cycle may occur in which insulin/leptin resistance and obesity aggravate one another. The vicious cycle is putatively fueled by continuously high insulin/leptin stimulation and fat storage, as a result of high intake of strongly insulin/leptin stimulating foods and energy. Both insulin and leptin normally function as satiety signals to the hypothalamus in the brain; however, insulin/leptin resistance may reduce this signal and therefore allow continued overfeeding despite large body fat stores. In addition, reduced leptin signaling to the brain may reduce leptin's normal effect to maintain an appropriately high metabolic rate.

There is debate about how and to what extent different dietary factors—e.g. intake of processed carbohydrates; total protein, fat, and carbohydrate intake; intake of saturated and trans fatty acids; and low intake of vitamins/minerals—contribute to the development of insulin- and leptin resistance. In any case, analogous to the way modern man-made pollution may potentially overwhelm the environment's ability to maintain 'homeostasis', the recent explosive introduction of high Glycemic Index and processed foods into the human diet may potentially overwhelm the body's ability to maintain homeostasis and health (as evidenced by the metabolic syndrome epidemic).

Vitamins and Minerals

Mineral and vitamin deficiency or excess may yield symptoms of diminishing health such as goiter, scurvy, osteoporosis, weak immune system, disorders of cell metabolism, certain forms of cancer, symptoms of premature aging, and poor psychological health (including eating disorders), among many others.

As of 2005, 12 vitamins and about the same number of minerals are recognized as essential nutrients, meaning that they must be consumed and absorbed—or, in the case of vitamin D, alternatively synthesized via UVB radiation—to prevent deficiency symptoms and death. Certain vitamin-like substances found in foods, such as carnitine, have also been found essential to survival and health, but these are not strictly "essential" to eat because the body can produce them from other compounds. Moreover, thousands of different phytochemicals have recently been discovered in food (particularly in fresh vegetables), which have many known and yet to be explored properties including antioxidant activity.

Antioxidants

Antioxidants are another recent discovery. As cellular metabolism/energy production requires oxygen, potentially damaging (e.g. mutation causing) compounds known as radical oxygen species or free radicals form as a result. For normal cellular maintenance, growth, and division, these free radicals must be sufficiently neutralized by antioxidant compounds. Some antioxidants are produced by the body with adequate precursors (glutathione, vitamin C). Those that the body cannot produce may only be obtained through the diet through direct sources (vitamins A, C, and K) or produced by the body from other compounds (Beta-carotene converted to vitamin A by the body, vitamin D synthesized from cholesterol by sunlight).

Some antioxidants are more effective than others at neutralizing different free radicals. Some cannot neutralize certain free radicals. Some cannot be present in certain areas of free radical development (vitamin A is fat-soluble and protects fat areas, vitamin C is water soluble and protects those areas).

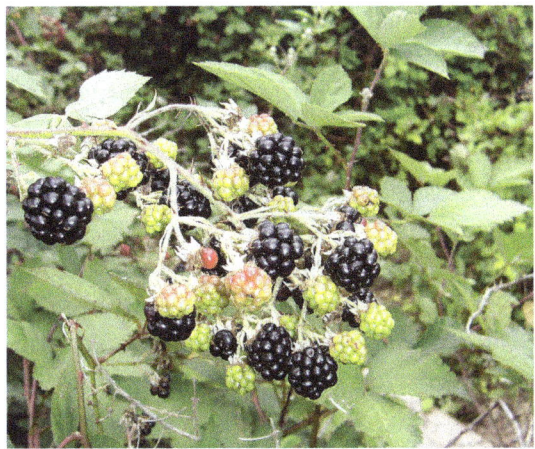

Blackberries are a source of polyphenol antioxidants.

When interacting with a free radical, some antioxidants produce a different free radical compound that is less dangerous or more dangerous than the previous compound. Having a variety of antioxidants allows any byproducts to be safely dealt with by more efficient antioxidants in neutralizing a free radical's butterfly effect.

Intestinal Bacterial Flora

It is now known that the human digestion system contains a population of a range of bacteria and yeast, such as bacteroides, L. acidophilus and E. coli, that are essential to digestion, and which are also affected by the food we eat. Bacteria in the gut fulfill a host of important functions for humans, including breaking down and aiding in the absorption of otherwise indigestible food; stimulating cell growth; repressing the growth of harmful bacteria, training the immune system to respond only to pathogens; and defending against some diseases.

Phytochemicals

A growing area of interest is the effect upon human health of trace chemicals, collectively called phytochemicals, nutrients typically found in edible plants, especially colorful fruits and vegetables. One of the principal classes of phytochemicals are polyphenol antioxidants, chemicals which are known to provide certain health benefits to the cardiovascular system and immune system. These chemicals are known to down-regulate the formation of reactive oxygen species, key chemicals in cardiovascular disease.

Perhaps the most rigorously tested phytochemical is zeaxanthin, a yellow-pigmented carotenoid present in many yellow and orange fruits and vegetables. Repeated studies have shown a strong correlation between ingestion of zeaxanthin and the prevention and treatment of age-related macular degeneration (AMD). Less rigorous studies have proposed a correlation between zeaxanthin intake and cataracts. A second carotenoid, lutein, has also been shown to lower the risk of contracting AMD. Both compounds have been observed to collect in the retina when ingested orally, and they serve to protect the rods and cones against the destructive effects of light.

Another caretenoid, beta-cryptoxanthin, appears to protect against chronic joint inflammatory diseases, such as arthritis. While the association between serum blood levels of beta-cryptoxanthin and substantially decreased joint disease has been established neither a convincing mechanism for such protection nor a cause-and-effect have been rigorously studied. Similarly, a red phyto-chemical, lycopene, has substantial credible evidence of negative association with development of prostate cancer.

The correlations between the ingestion of some phytochemicals and the prevention of disease are, in some cases, enormous in magnitude. For example, several studies have correlated high lev-els of zeaxanthin intake with roughly a 50 percent reduction in AMD. The difficulties in demon-strating causative properties and in applying the findings to human diet, however, are similarly enormous. The standard for rigorous proof of causation in medicine is the double-blind study, a time-consuming, difficult, and expensive process, especially in the case of preventative medicine. While new drugs must undergo such rigorous testing, pharmaceutical companies have a financial interest in funding rigorous testing and may recover the cost if the drug goes to market. No such commercial interest exists in studying chemicals that exist in orange juice and spinach, making funding for medical research difficult to obtain.

Even when the evidence is obtained, translating it to practical dietary advice can be difficult and counter-intuitive. Lutein, for example, occurs in many yellow and orange fruits and vegetables and protects the eyes against various diseases. However, it does not protect the eye nearly as well as zeaxanthin, and the presence of lutein in the retina will prevent zeaxanthin uptake. Addition-ally, evidence has shown that the lutein present in egg yolk is more readily absorbed than the lutein from vegetable sources, possibly because of fat solubility. As another example, lycopene is prevalent in tomatoes (and actually is the chemical that gives tomatoes their red color). It is more highly concentrated, however, in processed tomato products such as commercial pasta sauce, or tomato soup, than in fresh "healthy" tomatoes. Such sauces, however, tend to have high amounts of salt, sugar, other substances a person may wish or even need to avoid. The more we prepare food ourselves from fresh ingredients, the more knowledge and control we have about the undesirable additives.

Nutrition and Sports

Nutrition is very important for improving sports performance. Athletes need only slightly more protein than an average person, though strength-training athletes need more. Consuming a wide variety of protein sources, including plant-based sources, helps keep an overall health balance for the athlete.

Endurance, strength, and sprint athletes have different needs. Many athletes may require an in-creased caloric intake. Maintaining hydration during periods of physical exertion is an important element to good performance. While drinking too much water during activities can lead to physical discomfort, dehydration hinders an athlete's ability.

Sports Nutrition

Sports nutrition is the foundation of athletic success. It is a well-designed nutrition plan that al-lows active adults and athletes to perform at their best. It supplies the right food type, energy, nutrients, and fluids to keep the body well hydrated and functioning at peak levels. A sports nutrition diet may vary day to day, depending on specific energy demands.

Sports nutrition is unique to each person and is planned according to individual goals.

Goal of Sports Nutrition

Active adults and competitive athletes turn to sports nutrition to help them achieve their goals. Examples of individual goals could include gaining lean mass, improving body composition, or enhancing athletic performance. These sport-specific scenarios require differing nutritional programs. Research findings indicate the right food type, caloric intake, nutrient timing, fluids, and supplementation are essential and specific to each individual. The following are different states of training and competitive sport benefiting from sports nutrition:

Eating for Exercise/Athletic Performance

Training programs require a well-designed diet for active adults and competitive athletes. Research shows a balanced nutrition plan should include sufficient calories and healthy macronutrients to optimize athletic performance. The body will use carbohydrates or fats as the main energy source, depending on exercise intensity and duration. Inadequate caloric intake can impede athletic training and performance.

Active adults exercising three to four times weekly can usually meet nutritional needs through a normal healthy diet. Moderate to elite athletes performing intense training five to six times weekly will require significantly more nutrients to support energy demands.

Eating for Endurance

Endurance programs are defined as one to three hours per day of moderate to high-intensity exercise. High-energy intake in the form of carbohydrates is essential. According to research, target carbohydrate consumption for endurance athletes ranges from 6g to 10g per kilogram of body weight per day. Fat is a secondary source of energy used during long-duration training sessions. Endurance athletes are more at risk for dehydration. Replacing fluids and electrolytes lost through sweat are necessary for peak performance.

Eating for Strength

Resistance training programs are designed to gradually build the strength of skeletal muscle. Strength training is high-intensity work. It requires sufficient amounts of all macronutrients for muscle development. Protein intake is especially vital to increase and maintain lean body mass. Research indicates protein requirements can vary from 1.2 g to 3.1 g per kilogram of body weight per day.

Eating for Competition

Preparing for a competitive sport will vary in sports nutrition requirements. For example, strength athletes strive to increase lean mass and body size for their sport. Endurance runners focus on reduced body weight/fat for peak body function during their event. Athletic goals will determine the best sports nutrition strategy. Pre and post-workout meal planning are unique for each athlete and essential for optimal performance.

Sports Nutrition for Special Populations and Environments

Sports nutrition covers a wide spectrum of needs for athletes. Certain populations and environments require additional guidelines and information to enhance athletic performance:

- Vegetarian athlete: A vegetarian diet contains high intakes of plant proteins, fruits, vegetables, whole grains, and nuts. It can be nutritionally adequate, but insufficient evidence exists on long-term vegetarianism and athletic performance. Dietary assessments are recommended to avoid deficiencies and to ensure adequate nutrients to support athletic demands.

- High altitude: Specialized training and nutrition are required for athletes training at high altitude. Increasing red blood cells to carry more oxygen is essential. Iron-rich foods are an important component for this athlete as well. Increased risk of illness is indicated with chronic high altitude exposure. Foods high in antioxidants and protein are essential. Fluid requirements will vary per athlete, and hydration status should be individually monitored.

- Hot environments: Athletes competing in hot conditions are at greater risk of heat illness. Heat illness can have adverse health complications. Fluid and electrolyte balance is crucial for these athletes. Hydration strategies are required to maintain peak performance while exercising in the heat.

- Cold environments: Primary concerns for athletes exercising in the cold are adequate hydration and body temperature. Leaner athletes are at higher risk of hypothermia. Modifying caloric and carbohydrate intake are important for this athlete. Appropriate foods and fluids that withstand cold temperatures will promote optimal athletic performance.

Eating Disorders and Micronutrient Deficiencies in Sports Nutrition

Eating disorders in athletes are not uncommon. Many athletes are required to maintain lean bodies and low body weight and exhibit muscular development. Chronic competitive pressure can create psychological and physical stress of the athlete leading to disordered eating habits. Without proper counseling, adverse health effects may eventually develop. The most common eating disorders among athletes may include:

- Anorexia nervosa,

- Bulimia,

- Compulsive exercise disorder,

- Orthorexia.

Obviously, the nutritional needs of these individuals greatly differ from that of other active adults or athletes. Until someone with an eating disorder is considered well again, the primary focus should be put on treating and managing the eating disorder and consuming the nutrition needed to achieve and maintain good health, rather than athletic performance.

Micronutrient deficiencies are a concern for active adults and athletes. Exercise stresses important body functions where micronutrients are required. Additionally, athletes often restrict calories and certain food groups, which may potentially lead to deficiencies of essential micronutrients. Research indicates the most common micronutrient deficiencies include:

- Iron deficiency: Can impair muscle function and compromise athletic performance.

- Vitamin D deficiency: Can result in decreased bone strength and reduced muscle metabolic function.

- Calcium deficiency: Can impair the repair of bone tissue, decrease regulation of muscle contraction, and reduce nerve conduction.

Roles of a Sports Dietitian

Athletes and active adults are seeking guidance from sports professionals to enhance their athletic performance. Sports dietitians are increasingly hired to develop nutrition and fluid programs catered to the individual athlete or teams. A unique credential has been created for sports nutrition professionals: Board Certified Specialist in Sports Dietetics (CSSD). Sports dietitians should have knowledge in the following areas:

- Clinical nutrition.

- Nutrition science.

- Exercise physiology.

- Evidence-based research.

- Safe and effective nutrition assessments.

- Sports nutrition guidance.

- Counseling for health and athletic performance.

- Medical nutrition therapy.

- Design and management of effective nutrition strategies.

- Effective nutrition programming for health, fitness, and optimal physical performance.

Energy-yielding Nutrients

Carbohydrates

Carbohydrates, along with proteins and fats, are one of the main nutrients in our diets and provide the body with an essential source of energy. The body can store consumed carbohydrates as glycogen in the muscles and liver, but the storage capacity is limited (e.g. liver glycogen is depleted after about 28 hours of fasting). As exercise intensity increases, so does the reliance on carbohydrate fuel stores. Therefore keeping these stores adequately stocked is crucial for athletes who often need to perform at high exercise intensities (i.e., ≥70% of maximal aerobic power, VO_2 max). When body carbohydrate stores are inadequate they cannot meet the energy needs of the activities being performed. For an athlete, this can result in: fatigue, reduced training ability, impaired performance and reduced immune system function, which can impact on recovery.

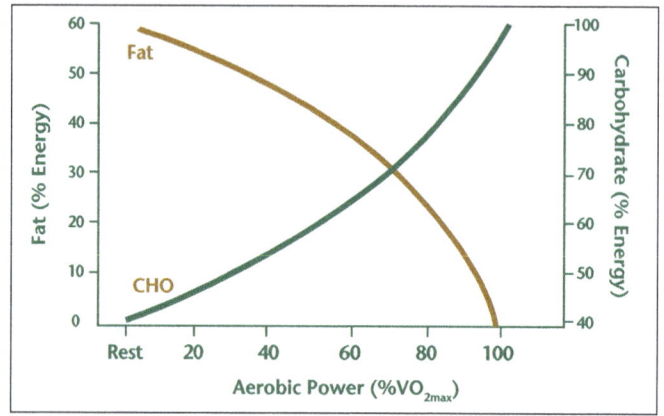

The relationship between the relative contribution of carbohydrate and fat utilization to energy expenditure as a function of relative power output. CHO denotes carbohydrate.

Carbohydrates Needed by Athletes

What is considered an adequate carbohydrate intake depends on the fuel requirements of an athlete's training and competition program, and also should take into account the frequency, duration and intensity of the activity being performed. Training and activity levels often change from day-to-day, week-to-week or month-to-month and an individual's carbohydrate intake should also fluctuate to reflect this. Figure provides some general guidance for daily carbohydrate intake goals for athletes based on exercise context and intensity. Generally, as the energetic demands of training or competition increase so does the dietary carbohydrate requirement, although these guidelines should be fine-tuned to take into account individual energy requirements, other training needs and athlete feedback.

Given the body's limited ability to store carbohydrates, for athletes seeking to optimize intense endurance performance during competition carbohydrate loading is often practiced, which typically involves consuming carbohydrate in the "High" or "Very High" range. Also, athletes preparing for training or competition are recommended to consume between 1-4 grams of carbohydrates per kilogram body mass in the 1-4 hours before exercise to ensure adequate fuelling. Performance can be further optimized by consuming carbohydrates during exercise with the amounts recommended dependent upon the nature of the activity. If training or competition is strenuous and lasts ~1 hour duration then small amounts of carbohydrates (15-30 grams per hour) can be considered. For endurance exercise or 'stop and go' sports such as half-marathon running or soccer lasting 1-2.5 hours, moderate amounts of carbohydrates are recommended (30-60 grams per hour) and for ultra-endurance exercise lasting over 2.5-3 hours such as marathon running or long bicycle events, larger amounts of carbohydrates (up to 90 grams per hour) could help to optimize performance. Finding carbohydrate sources that provide ~20-30 grams of carbohydrates per portion, such as whole foods (e.g. bananas) and carbohydrate-based sports drinks/gels/bars will enable athletes to simply tailor their intake by taking 1, 2 or 3 portions per hour depending on the nature of the exercise.

Type of Carbohydrates Consumed by Athletes

Athletes are generally advised to obtain their carbohydrates from a variety of foods including bread, cereals and grains, legumes, milk/alternatives, vegetables and fruits where the predominant carbohydrate, other than in milk and fruits, will be starch. Dietary surveys show sugars (mono- and disaccharides occurring naturally or added to food/drink in the diet) contribute 4-25% of total energy and 5-60% of carbohydrate intake in the diets of athletes. Clearly, sugars feature in the diets of athletes and given their high levels of physical activity and caloric needs, it seems reasonable that sugars can be regarded as one of a variety of options to help athletes achieve their specific carbohydrate-intake regimens as part of a normal pattern of food consumption.

Day-to-day carbohydrate intake can usually be obtained from normal food and drinks but specialty sports products such as sports drinks, energy gels and bars can be used to supplement food intake or as a convenient energy source during or for rapid recovery from intensive or prolonged training and competition. In these situations, the types of carbohydrate ingested can affect the speed at which energy is made available to the body and emphasis should be placed on consuming carbohydrates that can be rapidly absorbed and assimilated by the body, such as glucose, maltose and sucrose.

Table: Examples of Fast and Slow carbohydrate types.

'Fast' Carbohydrates	'Slow' Carbohydrates
Glucose	Fructose alone
Maltose	Galactose
Sucrose	Isomaltulose
Combined glucose and fructose	Starches rich in amylose
Maltodextrins	
Starches rich in amylopectin	

'Fast' and 'Slow' refer to the speed at which these carbohydrate types are generally digested, absorbed, and made available to the muscles and body for energy provision or storage during and after exercise.

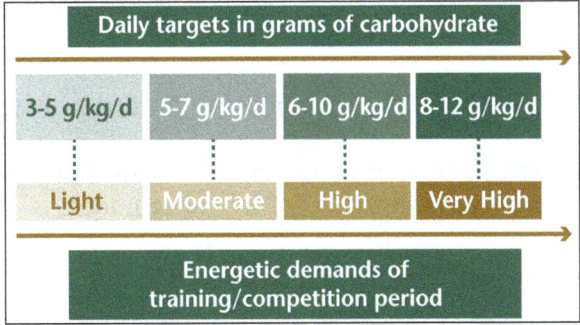

Figure above daily carbohydrate intake goals for athletes. Values expressed as grams of carbohydrate per kilogram body mass per day (g/kg/d). Light – low intensity or skill based activities;

Moderate – moderate exercise programme (~1 hour per day); High – endurance programme (e.g., moderate to high intensity exercise of 1-3 hours per day); Very high – extreme commitment (i.e., moderate to high intensity exercise of >4-5 hours per day).

Strategic Restriction of Carbohydrates and Exercise Adaptation

There is emerging evidence suggesting that the strategic restriction of carbohydrates during training sessions (such as occasionally training in the overnight-fasted state or training twice daily with limited carbohydrates consumed during recovery) may increase the activation of the molecular signals that trigger training adaptation in the exercise muscles. Although this adaptation may reduce the reliance on muscle glycogen as a fuel source during exercise, there is no clear evidence that this adaptation can eventually enhance exercise performance per se, and the impact/safety of repeated high-intensity training with low carbohydrate status needs to be further explored.

However, this does not mean that athletes should avoid carbohydrates in favour of high-fat diets, which seem unlikely to benefit most athletes engaged in high intensity sports. Given the critical role of carbohydrates in the optimization of sustained intense performance, it is still suggested by sports nutrition guidelines that key training sessions and competitions be undertaken with adequate carbohydrate fuel availability to meet energy needs and replenish glycogen stores.

For decades athletes have been using GI science for their sports preparation and recovery. Low GI foods have proven to extend endurance when eaten 1 – 2 hours before prolonged strenuous exercise.

Eating to Maximize your Sports Performance

Night before the Event

Planning ahead for a morning event, your evening meal should contain more carbohydrate than you would normally have. This is so you can fill up your glycogen stores. The carbohydrate should be low GI and the whole meal should be lower in fat, moderate in high quality protein and comfortable in quantity. Don't over eat.

Foods to Avoid Just before Exercise

The following foods may cause stomach discomfort due to their typically slow digestion:

- Any food high in fat.

- High fibre foods: White and some whole meal breads are acceptable – check the label.

- High protein: Make sure your protein intake is moderate to low, as it may also cause discomfort by slowing the rate of emptying from your stomach.

Breakfast on the Morning of the Event

This should be carbohydrate based, low fat and moderate in protein. Exactly what to eat, will depend on the time between breakfast and the start of the event. As with dinner you should only eat a comfortable amount of food, otherwise you will regret it.

During Event and Recovery Foods

During the event you should consume high GI carbohydrates – fluids like Gatorade and Powerade are often ideal.

One to 2 hrs after an event your food and fluid choices should be Low GI. Your body needs to replenish its glycogen stores, and delaying this replenishment can lead to fatigue. Replenishment of carbohydrate is generally 1 gram carbohydrate per 1kg body weight. So a 75 kg man needs 75 g carbohydrate for recovery after the event.

Fat

Fat is an important component of a diet designed to fuel exercise. One gram of dietary fat equals nine calories and one pound of stored fat provides approximately 3,600 calories of energy. This calorie density (the highest of all nutrients), along with our seemingly unlimited storage capacity for fat, makes it our largest reserve of energy. While these calories are less accessible to athletes performing quick, intense efforts like sprinting or weight lifting, fat is essential for longer, slower, lower intensity and endurance exercise, such as easy cycling and walking.

Everything we eat is made up of macro and micronutrients that are converted to energy inside the body, helping to fuel all of our bodily functions.

Dietary fat has been blamed for many health problems, but it is actually an essential nutrient for optimal health. Adipose tissue (stored fat) provides cushion and insulation to internal organs, covers the nerves, moves vitamins (A, D, E, and K) throughout the body, and is the largest reserve of stored energy available for activity.

Stored body fat is different from dietary fat. Body fat is only stored in the body when we consume more calories than we use, from any and all foods we eat, not just from dietary fats. There is an optimal level of body fat for health and for athletic activity.

Body's use of Fats

Fat provides the main fuel source for long-duration, low- to moderate-intensity exercise. Even during high-intensity exercise, where carbohydrate is the main fuel source, fat is needed to help access the stored carbohydrate (glycogen).

Using fat to fuel exercise, however, is dependent upon these important factors:

- Fat is slow to digest and be converted into a usable form of energy. (It can take up to six hours for this to occur.)

- After the body breaks down fat, it needs time to transport it to the working muscles before it can be used as energy.

- Converting stored body fat into energy takes a great deal of oxygen, so exercise intensity must decrease for this process to occur.

For these reasons, athletes need to carefully time when and how much fat they eat. In general, it's not a great idea to eat foods high in fat immediately before or during intense exercise. Aside from the fact that the workout will be done before the fat is available as usable energy, doing so can cause some uncomfortable gastrointestinal symptoms, such as nausea, vomiting, and diarrhea.

Dietary Fat

Dietary fat is frequently undervalued as a contributor to health and performance of athletes. Fat is an extremely important fuel for endurance exercise, along with carbohydrate, and some fat intake is required for optimal health. Dietary fat provides the essential fatty acids (EFA) that cannot be synthesized in the body.

The fat stores of the body are very large in comparison with carbohydrate stores. In some forms of exercise (e.g., prolonged cycling or running), carbohydrate depletion is possibly a cause of fatigue and depletion and can occur within 1 to 2 hours of strenuous exercise. The total amount of energy stored as glycogen in the muscles and liver has been estimated to be 8,000 kJ (2,000 kcal). Fat stores can contain more than 50 times the amount of energy contained in carbohydrate stores. A person with a body mass of 80 kg and 15% body fat has 12 kg of fat. Most of this fat is stored in subcutaneous adipose tissue, but some fat can also be found in muscle as intramuscular triacylglycerol (IMTG). In theory, fat stores could provide sufficient energy for a runner to run at least 1,300 km.

Table: Availability of substrates in the human body.

Substrate	Weight (kg)	Energy kJ (kcal)
Carbohydrates		
Plasma glucose	0.01	160 (40)
Liver glycogen	0.1	1,600 (400)
Muscle glycogen	0.4	6,400 (1,600)
Total (approximately)	0.51	8,000 (2,000)
Fat		
Plasma fatty acid	0.0004	16 (4)
Plasma triacylglycerols	0.004	160 (40)
Adipose tissue	12.0	430,000 (108,000)
Intramuscular triacylglycerols	0.3	11,000 (2,700)
Total (approximately)	12.3	442,000 (111,000)

Ideally, athletes would like to tap into their fat stores as much as possible and save the carbohydrate for later in a competition. Researchers, coaches, and athletes have therefore tried to devise nutritional strategies to enhance fat metabolism, spare carbohydrate stores, and thereby improve endurance performance. Understanding the effects of various nutritional strategies requires an understanding of fat metabolism and the factors that regulate fat oxidation during exercise.

Fat Metabolism during Exercise

FAs that are oxidized in the mitochondria of skeletal muscle during exercise are derived from various sources. The main two sources are adipose tissue and muscle triacylglycerols. A third fuel, plasma triacylglycerol may also be utilized, but the importance of this fuel is subject to debate. Triacylglycerols in adipose tissue are split into FAs and glycerol. The glycerol is released into the circulation, along with some of the FAs. A small percentage of FAs is not released into the circulation but is used to form new triacylglycerols within the adipose tissue, a process called reesterification. The other FAs are transported to the other tissues and taken up by skeletal muscle during exercise. Glycerol is transported to the liver, where it serves as a gluconeogenic substrate to form new glucose.

Besides the FAs in plasma, two other sources of FAs for oxidation in skeletal muscle are available. Circulating triacylglycerols (for example in a very low-density lipoprotein [VLDL]) can temporarily bind to lipoprotein lipase (LPL), which splits off FAs that can then be taken up by the muscle. A source of fat exists inside the muscle in the form of intramuscular triacylglycerol. These triacylglycerols are split by a hormone-sensitive lipase (HSL), and FAs are transported into the mitochondria for oxidation in the same way that FAs from plasma and plasma triacylglycerol are utilized.

Protein

Proteins are large molecules that our cells need to function properly. They consist of amino acids. The structure and function of our bodies depend on proteins. The regulation of the body's cells, tissues, and organs cannot happen without them.

Muscles, skin, bones, and other parts of the human body contain significant amounts of protein, including enzymes, hormones, and antibodies.

Proteins also work as neurotransmitters. Hemoglobin, a carrier of oxygen in the blood, is a protein.

Proteins are long chains of amino acids that form the basis of all life. They are like machines that make all living things, whether viruses, bacteria, butterflies, jellyfish, plants, or human function.

The human body consists of around 100 trillion cells. Each cell has thousands of different proteins. Together, these cause each cell to do its job. The proteins are like tiny machines inside the cell.

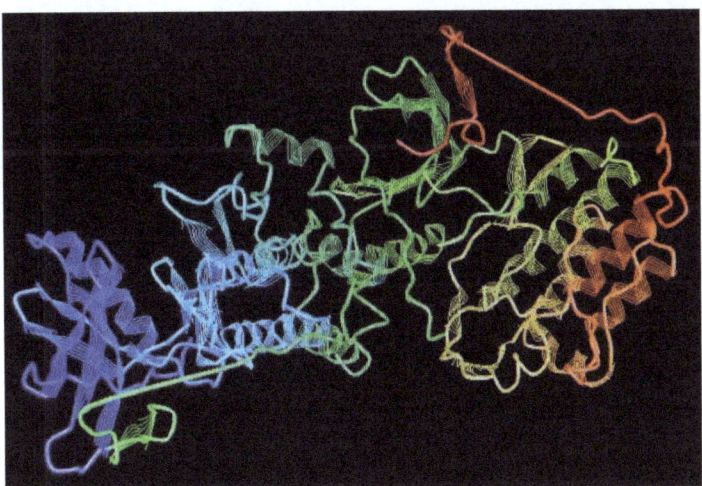

Protein molecules are essential for the functioning of every cell in the body. The body synthesizes some proteins foods we eat.

Amino Acids and Proteins

Protein consists of amino acids, and amino acids are the building blocks of protein. There are around 20 amino acids.

These 20 amino acids can be arranged in millions of different ways to create millions of different proteins, each with a specific function in the body. The structures differ according to the sequence in which the amino acids combine.

The 20 different amino acids that the body uses to synthesize proteins are: Alanine, arginine, asparagine, aspartic acid, cysteine, glutamic acid, glutamine, glycine, histidine, isoleucine, leucine, lysine, methionine, phenylalanine, proline, serine, threonine, tryptophan, tyrosine, and valine.

Amino acids are organic molecules that consist of carbon, hydrogen, oxygen, nitrogen, and sometimes sulfur.

It is the amino acids that synthesize proteins and other important compounds in the human body, such as creatine, peptide hormones, and some neurotransmitters.

Types of Protein

- Complete proteins: These foods contain all the essential amino acids. They mostly occur in animal foods, such as meat, dairy, and eggs.

- Incomplete proteins: These foods contain at least one essential amino acid, so there is a lack of balance in the proteins. Plant foods, such as peas, beans, and grains mostly contain incomplete protein.

- Complementary proteins: These refer to two or more foods containing incomplete proteins that people can combine to supply complete protein. Examples include rice and beans or bread with peanut butter.

Main Fucntions of Proteins

Proteins play a role in nearly every biological process, and their functions vary widely.

The main functions of proteins in the body are to build, strengthen and repair or replace things, such as tissue.

They can be:

- Structural, like collagen.

- Hormonal, like insulin.

- Carriers, for example, hemoglobin.

- Enzymes, such as amylase.

All of these are Proteins.

Keratin is a structural protein that strengthens protective coverings, such as hair. Collagen and elastin, too, have a structural function, and they also provide support for connective tissue.

Most enzymes are proteins and are catalysts, which means they speed up chemical reactions. They are necessary for respiration in human cells, for example, or photosynthesis in plants.

Sources

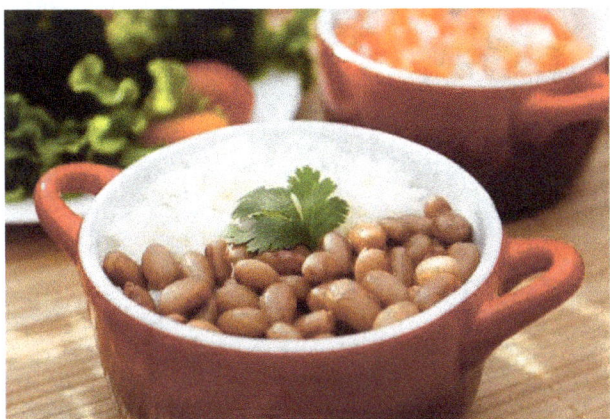

Rice and beans together provide complete protein.

Protein is one of the essential nutrients, or macronutrients, in the human diet, but not all the protein we eat converts into proteins in our body.

When people eat foods that contain amino acids, these amino acids make it possible for the body to create, or synthesize, proteins. If we do not consume some amino acids, we will not synthesize enough proteins for our bodies to function correctly.

There are also nine essential amino acids that the human body does not synthesize, so they must come from the diet.

All food proteins contain some of each amino acid, but in different proportions.

Gelatin is special in that it contains a high proportion of some amino acids but not the whole range.

The nine essential acids that the human body does not synthesize are: histidine, isoleucine, leucine, lysine, methionine, phenylalanine, threonine, tryptophan, and valine.

Foods that contain these nine essential acids in roughly equal proportions are called complete proteins. Complete proteins mainly come from animal sources, such as milk, meat, and eggs.

Soy and quinoa are vegetable sources of complete protein. Combining red beans or lentils with wholegrain rice or peanut butter with wholemeal bread also provides complete protein.

The body does not need all the essential amino acids at each meal, because it can utilize amino acids from recent meals to form complete proteins. If you have enough protein throughout the day, there is no risk of a deficiency.

In other words, the recommended nutrient is protein, but what we really need is amino acids.

Requirements

Exactly how much protein a person needs remains a matter of debate.

The FDA recommend that adults consume 50 grams of protein a day, as part of a 2,000-calorie diet. A person's daily value may be higher or lower depending on their calorie needs.

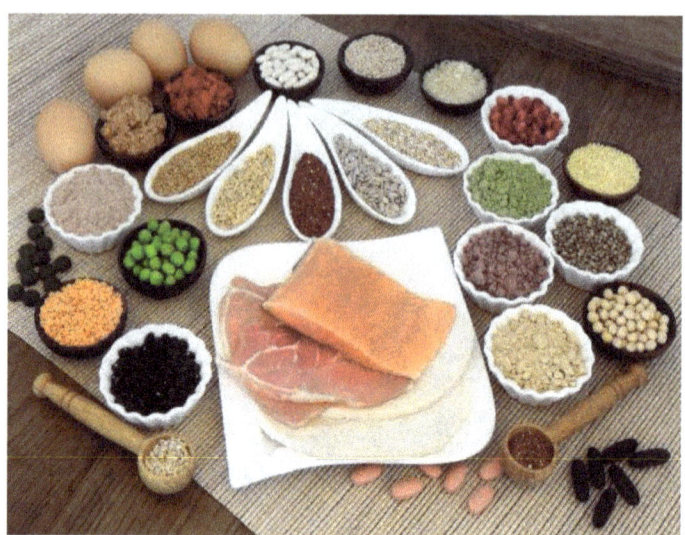

Protein foods do not have to be meat. Seafood,
eggs, pulses, and beans provide protein.

However, specifying exact amounts is difficult, because a range of factors, such as age, gender, activity level, and status, for example, pregnancy, play a role.

Other variables include the proportion of amino acids available in specific protein foods and the digestibility of individual amino acids. It also remains unclear how protein metabolism affects the need for protein intake.

The following foods will provide about 1 ounce of protein per serving listed below:

- One ounce lean meat, poultry, seafood.

- One ounce of meat, poultry, or seafood.

- One egg.

- One tablespoon of peanut butter.

- Half an ounce of nuts or seeds.

- One fourth of a cup of cooked beans or peas.

The USDA recommend consuming between 5 and 7 ounces of protein foods a day for most people over the age of 9 years.

Protein and Calories

Protein provides calories. One gram of protein contains 4 calories. One gram of fat has 9 calories.

The average American consumes around 16 percent of their calories from protein, whether of animal or plant origin.

It has been suggested that Americans obtain too many calories from protein, but now some experts are calling this a "misperception."

Protein and Weight Loss

Some diets recommend eating more protein in order to lose weight. Results of a review published in 2015 suggest that following a particular type of high-protein diet may encourage weight loss, but more work is needed to establish how to implement such a diet effectively.

Adding protein to an existing diet is unlikely to lead to weight loss, but replacing fat and sugar with protein might help. Replacing high-fiber foods — such as fruit, vegetables, and whole grains — with protein foods could have a negative effect.

People should consider their overall consumption and dietary habits when making this kind of change, and speak to a doctor before going ahead.

Protein Shakes and Foods

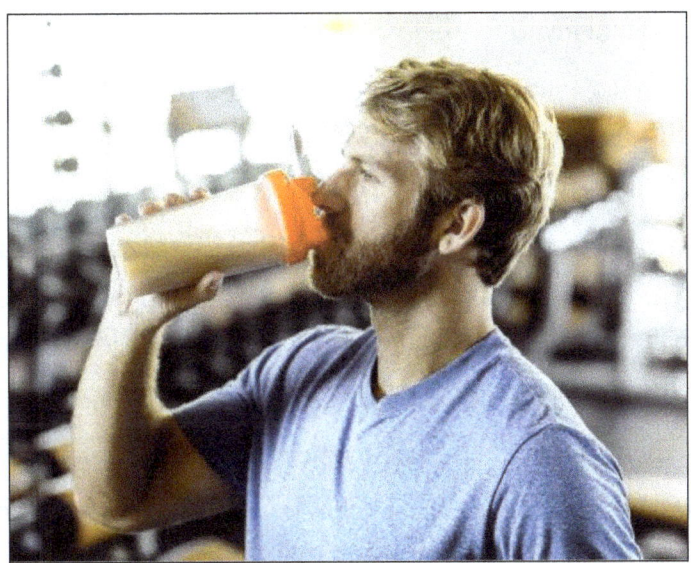

Protein shakes and supplements are popular with athletes, but people should use them with care.

Eating more protein may boost muscle strength and encourage a lean, fat-burning physique. However, this depends on the person's total food intake and activity levels.

Athletes and bodybuilders need to ensure they have enough protein to build and repair muscle, and this may be more than the minimum amount.

A wide range of protein supplements is currently available, many claiming to encourage weight loss and increase muscle mass and strength.

However, most athletes can get enough protein from a balanced diet without needing supplements. Some supplements may also contain banned or unhealthy substances. There is some evidence that too much protein may increase the risk of osteoporosis or kidney problems.

One study has indicated that whey protein may affect glucose metabolism and muscle protein synthesis. Other research concludes that at least one type of whey supplement can reduce body fat and preserve lean muscle when used in a reduced-calorie diet.

One investigation has found that whey protein enhanced performance in cyclists, and while another has suggested that it may lead to bone loss and osteoporosis, although this may also be due to other factors.

The UOM note that anyone using whey protein should not consume more than 1.2 grams for each 2.2 pounds of body weight.

In addition, as supplements, whey protein and similar products do not have FDA approval. This means is little or no control over their contents.

Anyone who is considering taking protein supplements for fitness purposes should speak to a doctor who specializes in sports medicine.

Protein Intake Guidelines

For most people, a varied and healthful diet will provide enough protein.

Increasing protein intake does not necessarily mean eating more steak. There are other choices that can help you ensure a healthful protein intake.

Here are some suggestions:

- Eat a variety of protein foods, choosing from fish, meat, soy, beans, tofu, nuts, seeds, and so on.
- Choose low-fat meat, poultry, and dairy products, and trim the fat from the meat. Opt for smaller portions and avoid processed meats, as they have added sodium.
- Use cooking methods that do not add extra fat, such as grilling.
- Check the ingredients in "protein bars,"as they can also be high in sugar.
- Opt for healthier versions of your usual favorites, for example, wholemeal rather than white bread and unsweetened peanut butter.
- Experiment with plant-based proteins, such as beans, lentils, and soy products.
- Choose nutrient-rich foods that provide other benefits, such as fiber.

Whether running sprints, swimming long distances or lifting weights, athletes expend more energy than the average person and their bodies need additional nutrients to recover from intense physical activity. Protein plays an important role in an athlete's diet as it helps repair and strengthen muscle tissue. High protein diets are popular among athletes — especially those seeking a leaner, more defined physique.

Overall Diet

While protein is critical in building muscle mass, more is not necessarily better. Simply eating large amounts of lean protein does not equate with a toned body.

When determining protein requirements for athletes, it's important to look at the athlete's overall diet. Athletes who consume diets adequate in carbohydrate and fat end up using less protein for energy than those who consume a higher protein diet. This means that protein can go toward building and maintaining lean body mass. Athletes need to ensure that they also are meeting needs for carbs and fat, not just protein.

Activity

Muscle growth happens only when exercise and diet are combined.

For example, research has shown that timing of protein intake plays a role. Eating high-quality protein (such as meat, fish, eggs, dairy or soy) within two hours after exercise — either by itself or with a carbohydrate — enhances muscle repair and growth.

Duration and intensity of the activity also are factors when it comes to protein needs.

Because they are building muscle, power athletes require a higher level of protein consumption than endurance athletes.

Recommendations

While athletes' protein needs are greater than that of non-athletes, they're not as high as commonly perceived. Researchers recommend 1.2 to 2.0 grams of protein per kilogram of body weight per day for athletes, depending on training. Protein intake should be spaced throughout the day and after workouts.

Most athletes can get the recommended amount of protein through food alone, without the use of supplements. Protein powders and supplements are great for convenience, but are not necessary, even for elite athletic performance. For example, protein powders can be useful when athletes need immediate protein right after a workout and don't have time for a meal.

Protein is essential for any athlete, particularly those actively training. It builds and repairs muscles, aids in recovery and helps your muscles adapt fully in response to your training. Unlike glucose, which your body can synthesize even if you do not eat carbohydrates, your body cannot manufacture protein from other sources. Without enough protein, your body will start breaking down muscle to get the amino acids it needs to function.

Proteins are complex molecules formed by smaller sub-units called amino acids. There are 20 known amino acids, each belonging to one of three groups. Essential amino acids include 10 amino acids that your body cannot make on its own. Non-essential amino acids are the amino acids you can synthesize either from essential amino acids or from protein. The third group, the conditional amino acids, contains amino acids that are usually non-essential, but can become essential when your body is under stress.

For a body to get the amount of amino acids it requires each day, all adults must consume at least 0.8 grams of protein per kilogram of body weight. Bodybuilders and athletes who are actively training, must consume at least 1.2 to 2.0 grams of protein per kilogram of body weight per day, depending on training.

Keep in mind, some sources of protein are better than others. The best dietary protein sources offer a balanced profile of amino acids, a high concentration of protein, additional nutrients and healthy amounts of fats.

Wild Fish

Fish packs a ton of protein in a low calorie, nutritious package. Three ounces of wild salmon, for example, has 19 grams of protein with only 175 calories. Fish also provides important omega-3s for your heart and brain. Whenever possible, look for wild caught fish. Farm raised fish are not fed a natural diet, are often sick and do not have the same concentration of omega-3s as wild caught fish.

Eggs

Rich in thiamine, riboflavin, pantothenic acid, folic acid, vitamin B12, biotin, vitamin D, vitamin E and phosphorus, eggs are a powerhouse of protein and nutrients. They are also easy to digest and quick to prepare. Look for whole, organic, cage-free eggs which will be far more nutrient-rich. Lastly, make sure to include the egg yolks in your diet. The yolk contains the concentration of vitamins, minerals, antioxidants and omega-3 fatty acids that will keep your brain and body strong.

Chicken

Chicken contains all essential amino acids and is easy to digest. A 100g serving contains 27 g of protein and 239 calories. When buying chicken, look for chicken that was raised in cage-free, humane conditions and was fed a nutrient-dense, variable diet.

Grass-fed Beef

Grass-fed beef offers cleaner, more flavorful, more nutrient-rich meat than grain-fed beef. It is packed with zinc, iron and all essential amino acids.

Whey Protein

The second most abundant protein derived from milk, whey protein is found primarily in meal-replacement powders and protein powders. Whey contains all the essential amino acids and is high in the branched-chain amino acids: leucine, isoleucine and valine. It is also high in glutamine which boosts immune and muscle recovery. When buying whey, make sure it comes from cows that are grass-fed an organic diet and free from hormones.

Almonds

Almonds serve as a great source of protein and energy, as well as act as an anti-inflammatory. They provide vitamin E, fiber and healthy fat.

Greek Yogurt

Low in sugar, relatively high in protein and rich in healthy fat, organic Greek yogurt is a great addition to a balanced diet.

Strength and endurance exercise go a long way in athletic training, but nothing can replace nutrition. Without protein, muscles deteriorate, energy declines and recovery slows. Fortunately, an athlete can achieve the recommended protein amounts through diet alone.

Energy Expenditure

The energy that human body requires to maintain its organic and vital functions is obtained by the oxidation of macronutrients from foods. Energy expenditure (EE) can be considered a process of energy production from energy substrates (carbohydrates, lipids, proteins and alcohol) combustion, in which there is an oxygen consumption (O_2) and carbon dioxide production (CO_2). Part of this chemical energy is lost as heat and in urine, and the remain energy is stored in high-energy molecules known as adenosine triphosphates (ATPs). Total energy expenditure (TEE) is the energy required by the organism daily and it is determined by the sum of 3 components: basal energy expenditure (BEE), dietinduced thermogenesis (DIT) and physical activity (PA). There are several methods for EE measurementsuch as indirect calorimetry (IC) and direct calorimetry (DC), bioelectrical impedance (BIA), doubly labeled water (DLW), predictive equations, and others. The EE determination is important to adjust the individuals' nutritional offer, and must consider the demand of energy for physical activity and specific health conditions. Most of these methods have been widely used in human studies for different clinical applications (enteral and parenteral nutrition, obesity and others). However, there is no consensus about the applicability of some of them due to different results from literature.

Components of Total Energy Expenditure

Basal Energy Expenditure

The BEE is the amount of calories spent per minute or per hour which can be extrapolated to 24 hours, it also represents the minimal energy required for body vital function maintenance. The BEE is one of the most important physiological information in clinical and epidemiological nutritional studies, since it is used to determine the energy requirement of an individual or population.

The BEE contributes for 60% to 70% of daily energy requirement for most sedentary individuals and nearly 50% for those physically active. Its determination is useful to compare the energy metabolism between individuals.

This component of TEE must be measured under standardized ambient conditions such as controlled temperature and humidity. Subject must be at complete rest after at least 8 hours of sleep and after a 12-14 hour overnight fast. Also, during the measurement, subject must be kept fully awake, lied down quietly, completely relaxed and breathing normally. The value obtained is extrapolated to the 24 hours of the day and, therefore, is referred to basal with minimal influence of DIT and PA in the TEE. However, the measurement of BEE requires the subject to sleep overnight in the metabolic unit. Thus, instead of BEE, the resting energy expenditure (REE) is usually measured, since there is little difference between them.

Many individual factors may affect BEE, such as ethnicity, weight, lean body mass, age, smoking habits, PA, diet, menstrual period and fasting. Room's conditions (temperature, noise and time of resting) and technical factors related to the equipments used may also affect the BEE measurement. For example, the metabolic monitor must be heated and stabilized 30 minutes before each determination and the gas analyzers must be calibrated with a known gas concentration and perio dically validated with the use of methanol flame. Other factors which may also affect BEE at different levels would be thyroid and sexual hormones; growth; fever; sleep; metabolic stress; diseases; and others.

Resting Energy Expenditure

The REE is a component of EE that is also measured by indirect calorimetry (IC). It can be 3-10% higher than BEE due to DIT and the influence of most recent PA.

The procedures for measuring REE are very similar to those for BEE. The greatest difference between them is that in REE estimation the subjects have to be resting and fasting for shorter time, at least 30-minute rest and 3- hour fasting.

Thermic Effect of Food or Diet-induced Thermogenesis

Diet-induced thermogenesis (DIT) is the EE component related to the energy required for the digestion, absorption, usage and storage of nutrients after food intake. The DIT represents 5% to 15% of the TEE, and plays an important role in the regulation of energy balance and of body weight. The thermic effect of food on TEE varies according to the type of macronutrient intake: 0-3% for lipids, 5-10% for carbohydrates and 20-30% for proteins.

DIT is higher for proteins because their synthesis requires at least four high-energy phosphate bonds (ATP) per amino acid incorporated into a protein molecule, with the dispent of 0,75 kcal/g of synthesized protein, and the high metabolic cost of ureogenesis and gluconeogenesis. DIT can be divided into two distinct phases: the cephalic and the gastrointestinal phases. The first one is related to sympathetic nervous system action which is activated by food sensory properties, while the second is characterized by ATP consumption during the absorption and utilization of nutrients. There are some factors that may influence and modulate DIT, such as the stimulus to the autonomic nervous system, hormones, diet palatability, PA, body composition, adiposity, and the most important, diet composition.

Physical Activity (PA)

Physical activity (PA) represents the thermic effect of any movement that exceeds BEE, which have a great variability inter and intra individual. In active individuals, the energy required for PA can corresponds as one to two times the basal energy expenditure while in sedentary individuals it can represent less than half of the BEE.

Available Methods for Determination of Energy Expenditure

There are many methods for determining EE, but there is no consensus about which is the most accurate one for specific individuals or populations.

Direct Calorimetry

The directly determination of EE represents the measurement of heat exchange between body and environment. This method measures the sensible heat released by the body, as well as the water steam released through respiration and skin. It requires an isolation chamber, hermetically sealed, highly sophisticated and large enough to allow some degree of activity. Although it is considered a gold standard method, it is not widely used due to its high complexity and cost, moreover, it requires the individual a confinement of 24 hours or more.

Respiratory Indirect Calorimetry

Respiratory indirect calorimetry, or only indirect calorimetry (IC) as it is often known by most authors, is a noninvasive and very accurate method which has an error lower than 1%. It has high reproducibility and has being considered a gold standard method. This method allows estimating BEE and REE, and also allows identifying which energy substrates is predominantly being metabolized by body in a specific moment. It is based on the indirect measure of the heat expended by nutrients oxidation, which is estimated by monitoring oxygen consumption (O_2)and carbon dioxide production (CO_2) for a certain period of time.

The calorimeter has a gas collector that adapts to subject, a canopy and a system that measures the volume and concentrations of O_2 and CO_2 minute by minute. Through a unidirectional valve located in the ventilated canopy, the calorimeter collect and quantify the volume and concentration of O_2 inspired and of CO_2 expired by the subject. After meeting the volu mes, EE is calculated by the Weir formula and results are displayed in a software attached to the system.

The procedures for using IC requires the same standardized protocol for determining BEE and REE, which includes environmental, individual, and technical aspects. One advantage of using this method is the fact that it allows a short term measurement due to the scarce O_2 body reservoirs and the limited capacity of body of anaerobic ATP synthesis. However, it is costly, relatively complex and requires trained personnel for its correct use.

Circulatory Indirect Calorimetry (CIC) or Fick Principle

REE can also be measured by CIC which is a practical and simple method. The CIC is commonly used to monitor O_2 consumption and EE when an intensive care unit (ICU) does not have IC and patients' nutritional support must be done with caution.

This method is based on a thermo dilution technique that requires the insertion of a catheter into the pulmonary artery for estimating cardiac output. Besides, the use of this catheter allows analyzing the arterial and venous blood gasometry which is based on the measurement of the serum hemoglobin concentration and its O_2 saturation. It is possible to calculate O_2 consumption through the artero-venous difference of the O_2 content multiplied by the cardiac output. Thus, REE can be estimated based on the Fick equation. However CIC requires a surgical procedure to insert the catheter, so that this method should only be used when critical patients has already had a catheter inserted in their artery for hemodynamic control.

Similarly to other method, CIC also has some limitations as it is invasive and the usage of catheters may contribute for complications. Furthermore, it is based on instantaneous measures, thus extreme values of cardiac output decrease the specificity of thermo dilution, as well as the omission of the O_2 dissolved in the plasma and exclusion of the pulmonary O_2 mixed to the O_2 coming from other organs can decrease its specificity.

Table: Advantages and limitations of assessment methods of energy expenditure.

Method	Advantages	Limitations
Direct calorimetry	Highly sophisticated method, considered a gold standard for measuring the total energy expenditure, allows the subject some degree of activity.	High complexity method, high cost and requires the confinement of the subject for 24 hours or more.
Indirect calorimetry	This method is considered a gold standard for measuring REE and BEE. It is a non-invasive method, reasonably accurate and has a high reproducibility. It also allows to quantify and to identify energy substrates oxidation. Allows short-term measurements of EE.	High cost, relatively complex. Requires trained personnel for its correct use.
Circulatory indirect calorimetry	Practical and simple method. It can be used with caution when there is no other way to assess EE in critically ill patients who have already have a thermo-dilution catheter inserted.	It is Invasive. The use of the catheter may contribute to metabolic complications. It is based on instantaneous measurements. It is not equivalent to CI because it underestimates the REE.
Double labeled water	This is a gold standard method which accuracy is 97-99% compared to CI. It measures precisely the TEE in free living subjects and because it uses deuterium (H2) and oxygen-18 (O18), it is a safe method.	It is costly and requires sophisticated equipments as well as trained personnel. It does not provide the information of energy expedited on physica activity neither it gives the information about the substrates oxidation.
Bioelectrical impedance analysis	This is an affordable and non-invasive method. It quickly estimates the REE based on its estimation of body compartments including the body fluid distribution considering intra and extracellular spaces.	Several factors may influence its results such as hydration state of the subject, prandial/fasting state, exercises, diuretics use, menstrual period, age, ethnicity, body shape or healthy and nutritional condition.
Sensor of heat and movement	Easy and practical use device that estimates EE.	Studies indicate that the device needs adjusts, especially the equations for obese subjects.
Physical activities records	• Low cost method that estimates EE from an extremely detailed registry off all physical activity perform daily. • Wide variety of types of activities listed. The list is frequently updated which allows the inclusion or the correction of typical activities from specific regions or country.	• The comparison of results between different studies is limited due to various existing codes for activities. • The estimated EE does not take into account inter-individual differences which may affect the energetic cost of a movement.
Dietary questionnaires	Simple and affordable method. It can be viable if properly used.	• Subjects can underreport their food intake, which will reduce de accuracy of the method. • This method is valid only for subjects with stable weight, so in a energy balance equilibrium. • Bias can occur because of interferences from the interviewer as well as bias inherent in the chosen method.
Predictive equations	Simple, fast and affordable method. It can be viable if properly used.	It can overestimate or underestimate the GEB GET of subjects of the same population.

Raurish and Ibanez evaluated the EE of 15 critically ill patients on mechanical ventilation through the IC and CIC, and they found no significant difference between these two methods. Despite the lower reproducibility of Fick compared to IC, they concluded that both methods can be used considering the clinical point of view. However, Ogawa et al. evaluated the EE of 40 critically ill patients in ICU and although they did not find a significant difference between IC and CIC, the use of Fick equation on CIC underestimated the absolute values. Similarly, in another study with 36 patients on mechanical ventilation and parenteral nutrition, the Fick equation underestimated significantly REE compared to IC, and these methods had a poor correlation ($r = 0.31$).

The CIC can be a useful tool if used with caution when there is no other way to assess the EE of critically ill patients who already have a thermo dilution catheter inserted. However, it is important to emphasize that this method is not equivalent to IC, because it underestimates REE values.

Doubly Labeled Water

The DLW is an accurate and precise method for measuring TEE of subjects who are not in confinement, and with no change their routine, it also useful for measuring TEE over some days or weeks. It is considered safe because uses deuterium (H^2) and oxygen-18 (O^{18}), nonradioactive elements which are naturally found in human body. The DLW accuracy is 97-99% compared to IC, and it is also considered a gold standard.

This method is based on the principle of isotope dilution. Subject ingests those elements at a known concentration and volume (C_1 and V_1) that diffuses throughout the body fluid (which has a different volu - me (V_2), and the new concentration (C_2) can be calculated by the formula $C_1 \times V_1 = C_2 \times V_2$. Thus, the DLW method considers that the O_2 turnover is determined by the body water flow and the inspired O_2 and expired CO_2, while the H_2 turnover is determined exclusively by the water flow through the body.

To measure the total body water, a pre-established volume and concentration of the H^2 and O^{18} isotope is orally administered, which diffuses throughout the body over 2 to 6 hours. As the energy is spent by the body, CO_2 and water are produced. The CO_2 is eliminated by the lungs, and the water, by lungs, skin and urine. The H^2 and O^{18} disappearance rate is determined by measuring repeatedly their concentrations in the body fluids (saliva, urine or blood). The difference between the disappearance rate of the two isotopes is used to estimate the CO_2 production rate and, thus, determine the EE, based on the equation of Weir.

Many studies have used DLW to validate other methods. However, this method is expensive, requires sophisticated equipments and trained personnel. Besides, it does not provide information of performed physical activity and substrate oxidation.

Bioelectrical Impedance Analysis (BIA)

BIA is a fast and noninvasive method that estimates body composition, including the distribution of body fluids of intra and extracellular spaces. It also estimates REE by predictive equations based on the lean body mass.

This method can be performed by devices with 2, 4 or 8 electrodes. It is based on the principle that tissues have different electrical proprieties such as large at small opposition to the flow of an electric current. Lean tissues have a high conductivity of electric current, due to the large amount of water and electrolytes. On the other hand, adipose tissue (fat body mass), bones and skin have low conductivity. This method mesures the level of resistance (measure of pure opposition to the electric current flow through the body) and reactance (opposition to the electric current flow caused by the capacitance produced by the cell membrane) of the body to a low intensity electric current. By doing so, the analyzer evaluates the total body water, assuming a constant hydration, predicts the amount of lean body mass and estimates REE based on this value.

The usage of BIA has some limitations related to individuals' hydration status. In case of hyperhydration or fluid retention, both lean body mass and REE will be overestimated. Besides, other factors may affect the results of BIA, such as diet, physical activity, use of diuretics, menstrual period, age, ethnic group, body shape or clinical and nutritional status. Korth et al. reported that EE estimation through equations based on the lean body mass may be more accurate than those that the estimation is mainly based on body weight, assuming that the lean body mass is the responsible for 60-70% of the REE variation.

Strain et al. studied severe obese adults and evaluated body composition by BIA and DLW, and EE by BIA and IC. The BIA and DLW methods showed high correlation (r = 0,92) for estimation of total body water and lean body mass, as well as equivalence by the Bland and Altman analysis. The REE values obtained by BIA and IC did not differ significantly, and showed high correlation (r = 0.88). Therefore, those authors suggested the use of bipolar BIA to estimate the body composition and REE of obese individuals. However, for normal weight and overweight individuals, Oliveira et al. found that comparing to IC, tetrapolar BIA significantly underestimated the BEE of healthy women, but the same did not occur to men.

Korth et al. evaluated lean body mass of 104 normal weight adults by different methods, and the EE by IC and equations which consider body composition. Lean body mass estimated by those several methods did not differ significantly, and all methods were highly correlated (r = 0.95-0.99). The variations observed for REE estimated by equations were better explained by the differences on their mathematical model and data that used in their determination than the method for body composition itself. Those authors conclude that there is no advantage in using a more accurate method for body composition when the objective is to estimate the EE based on the lean body mass. But it is important to use the appropriate equation for a specific population.

The REE estimation by BIA is valid for clinical practice, when the right protocol for this method is respected, mainly because it is a noninvasive and less expensive when compared to IC.

Sensor of Heat and Movement

The heat and movement sensor SenseWear Pro 2 Armband is a practical device recently developed. This device estimates the EE through equations developed by the manufacturer which considers several parameters (heat flow, accelerometer, galvanic skin response, skin temperature, temperature close to the body) and characteristics of each subject (sex, age, height, body weight, right-handed or left-handed and smoker and nonsmoker).

St-Onge et al. measured the TEE and EE considering physical activity of individuals in free-living conditions, by using Armband and compared the results with the DLW technique. The authors observed a slight underestimation in the TEE (117 kcal/day) compared to the DLW, and a good correlation between these methods (r = 0.81; P < 0.01). On the other hand, the EE considering physical activity estimated by Armband, were less accurate, showing a 218 kcal/day underestimation compared to the DLW and both had a correlation of 46% (P < 0.01). However, it is well known that EE considering physical activity measured by DLW is obtained from a derived value. So that there is a potential error associated with the addition or subtraction of other components (BEE and DIT). Therefore, it is unclear if the lower accuracy in the determination of the EE considering physical activity is due to a limitation of Armband to capture different types of physical activity, or the inaccuracy of DLW for physical activity.

Papazouglou et al. tested the reliability and validity of the SenseWear Pro 2 Armband, during rest and exercise compared to the IC in obese people. They found poor accuracy of Armband in the measurement of the EE, both at rest and in exercise, mainly in obese with higher EE values. According to those authors, it is necessary to incorporate new algorithms specific for obesity to the software in order to improve its accuracy. Similarly, a low concordance between these two methods to estimate the REE was found by Bertoli et al. in a study carried out in 169 adults of which 48% were obese. The device significantly overestimated the REE compared to IC for both gender. Through the Bland Altman analysis, the authors concluded that these methods are not equivalent. Thus, until this moment, studies showed that the sensor of heat and movement device needs adjustments for estimating more accurately the EE.

Physical Activity Records

Physical activity records estimates EE from a very detailed report of all physical activities (PA) performed daily. Most of the times, it is considered a complementary method, due to its subjectivity.

The PA data are encoded according to its type and intensity and is used to describe a population physical activity pattern and to study its determinants. Moreover, through these records it is possible to investigate the relationships between PA, health and disease. It also can be used to evaluated the contribution of several types of PA to TEE, providing additional categories for the type of activities routinely performed.

Among the lists of codes that exist, there is The Compendium of Physical Activity, published in 1993. The compendium consists of five-digit codes that represent specific activities carried out in several situations with their respective levels of intensity expressed in metabolic equivalent units (METs).

The EE is expressed in $kcal.kg^{-1}$ of body $weight.h^{-1}$; $kcal.min^{-1}$; $kcal.h^{-1}$ or $kcal.24 h^{-1}$. It is possible to estimate individual EE (kcal) by multiplying body weight (kg) by the duration of the PA (minutes) and by MET value obtained in the compendium.

Generally, it is assumed that the REE of any individual is equal to 1 MET. Therefore, in this case, the EE with physical activities must be expressed in resting METs. The steps for calculating EE is showed below:

- 1,000 ml O2 = 5 kcal.

- 200 ml O_2 = 1 kcal.

- 1 MET = 3.5 mL O_2/kg/min (VO_2 at rest).

- 3.5 mL O_2 /kg /min: 200 ml O_2 = 0.0175/kg/min or.

- Equation: 0.0175 × weight (kg) × METs = kcal/min.

The O_2 consumption varies with age resulting in different values of METs. For example, for teenagers between 16 and 17 years, 1 MET corresponds to 4.0 mL O_2 /kg/min. For individuals between 12 and 13 years of age, 1 MET corresponds to 4.58 mL O_2 /kg/min and for children below 5 years of age is 7.0 mL O_2 /kg/min.

Conway et al., in a study with 24 adult men with Body Mass Index (BMI) of 25. 1 ± 0, 5 kg/m², compared the TEE measured by DLW, with 7-day physical activities records and with a 7-day physical activity recalls. They found a good correlation between the physical activity records and the DLW, while the physical activities recalls had a limited application in estimating daily energy due to its overestimation of 30,6%.

However, the major problem of this method is that different authors use different codes for the same type and intensity of physical activities. Although there are similarities in some publications, the comparison of results among the several studies is limited. Another important limitation is that EE estimated through this method does not consider the individuals' differences that can influence the energy cost of the movement. Therefore, a correction factor would be necessary for individual adjustments considering gender, age, physiological status, body composition, and others, which does not exist yet. On the other hand, the major advantage of using this method is the wide variety of activities listed that have constant updates because of studies that include this method, which allow the inclusion or correction of specific activities to a particular region or country.

Energy Balance

"Energy balance" is the relationship between "energy in" (food calories taken into the body through food and drink) and "energy out" (calories being used in the body for our daily energy requirements).

This relationship, which is defined by the laws of thermodynamics, dictates whether weight is lost, gained, or remains the same.

According to these laws, energy is never really created and it's never really destroyed. Rather, energy is transferred between entities.

We convert potential energy that's stored within our food (measured in Calories or kcals) into three major "destinations": work, heat and storage.

The average number of available calories per person in the US is increasing. In general, there is more "energy in".

When it comes to "energy out," the body's energy needs include the amount of energy required for maintenance at rest, physical activity and movement, and for food digestion, absorption, and transport.

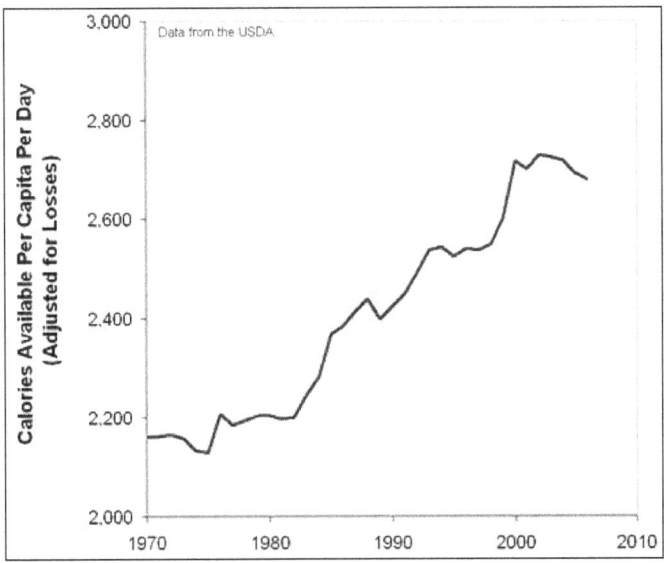

We can estimate our energy needs by measuring the amount of oxygen we consume. We eat, we digest, we absorb, we circulate, we store, we transfer energy, we burn the energy, and then we repeat.

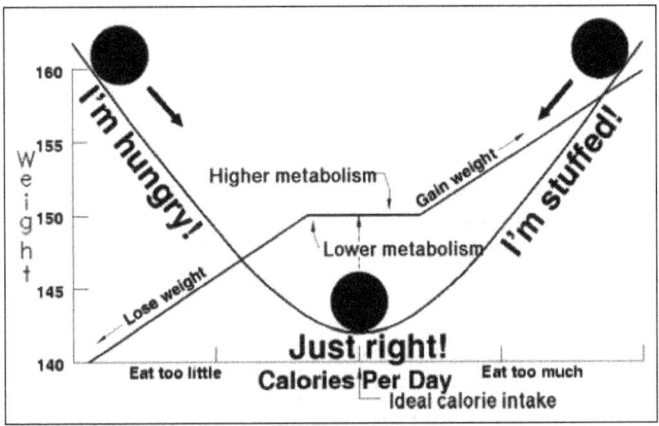

Importance of Energy Balance

There's a lot more to energy balance than a change in body weight.

Energy balance also has to do with what's going on in your cells. When you're in a positive energy balance (more in than out) and when you're in a negative energy balance (more out than in), everything from your metabolism, to your hormonal balance, to your mood is impacted.

Negative Energy Balance

A severe negative energy balance can lead to a decline in metabolism, decreases in bone mass, reductions in thyroid hormones, reductions in testosterone levels, an inability to concentrate, and a reduction in physical performance.

Yet a negative energy balance does lead to weight loss. The body detects an energy "deficit" and fat reserves are called upon to make up the difference.

The body doesn't know the difference between a strict diet monitored by a physician and simply running out of food. The body just knows it isn't getting enough energy, so it will begin to slow down (or shut down) all "non-survival" functions.

Positive Energy Balance

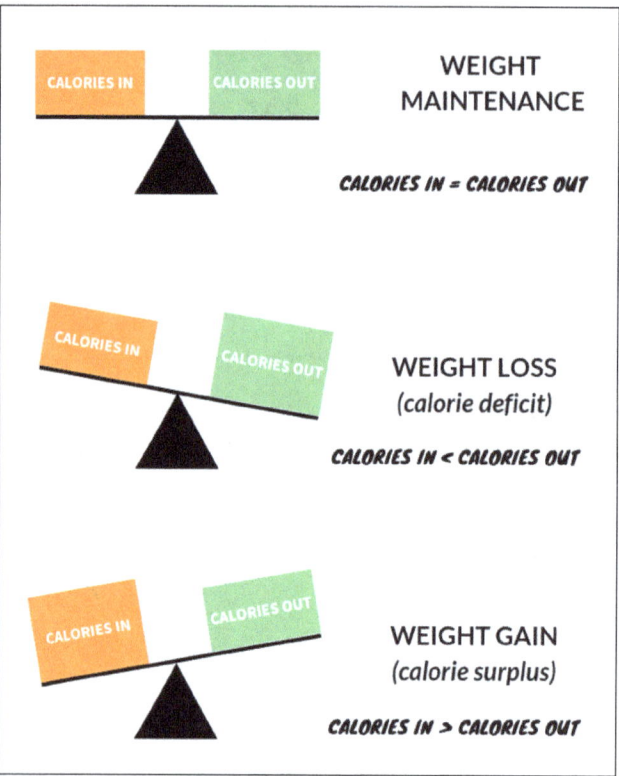

Overfeeding (and under exercising) has its own ramifications not only in terms of weight gain but in terms of health and cellular fitness. With too much overfeeding, plaques can build up in arteries, the blood pressure and cholesterol in our body can increase, we can become insulin resistant and suffer from diabetes, we can increase our risk for certain cancers, and so on.

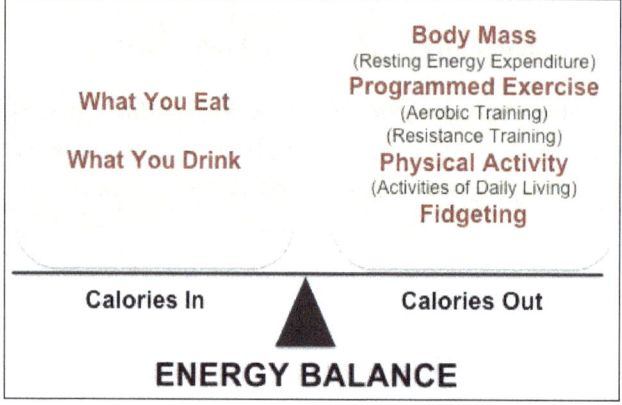

The relationship between the amount of Calories we eat in the diet and the amount of energy we use in the body determines our body weight and overall health.

The body is highly adaptable to a variety of energy intakes/outputs. It must be adaptable in order to survive. Therefore, mechanisms are in place to ensure stable energy transfer regardless of whether energy imbalances exist.

The standard view of energy balance doesn't offer consistent explanations for body composition changes.

This is because calorie restriction or over-consumption without a "metabolic intervention" (such as exercise or drugs) is likely to produce equal losses in lean mass and fat mass with restriction or equal gains in lean mass and fat mass with overfeeding.

People will likely end up as smaller or larger versions of the same shape. They'll lose muscle along with fat.

Both sides of the energy balance equation are complex and the interrelationships determine body composition and health outcomes.

Overall lifestyle habits help to properly control energy balance, and when properly controlled, excessive swings in either direction (positive or negative) are prevented and the body can either lose fat or gain lean mass in a healthy way.

Factors that affect Energy in

- Calorie intake.
- Energy digested and absorbed (90-99%).

Factors that Affect Energy Out

Work

- Physical work (exercise and activity).

Heat

- Heat produced with physical work.
- Heat produced via the thermic effect of food (TEF).
- Heat produced by resting metabolism.
- Heat produced: adipose creation.
- Heat produced: adipose thermoregulation.

Storage

- Efficiency of work.
- Efficiency of food metabolism.
- Energy stored in adipose tissue.

Ideal Diet for a Sports Person

Sports is very demanding on the body. A wicketkeeper in Cricket does a minimum of 540 squats in a single day of a test match, Tennis involves the repetitive movement of wrists; Golf requires a lot of bending & lifting and during intense training sessions body's muscle work rate can increase more than 25 times. An athlete's body is a machine and in order to make this machine work at its peak and prevent injury, they need to put in the right fuel (food).

Right foods taken in the right quantity at the right time have a huge impact on improving sports performance. A healthy diet plan helps athletes to train harder, recover faster and lessens the probability of injury occurrence. Athletes require extra calories to fuel their activities & provide strength to muscle and bones. High-level endurance athletes require 3000-6000 calories/day; those playing team sports require 4000-5000 calories/day. The calorie intake has to be planned meticulously and in correct proportion according to their sport and training across 6-9 meals throughout the day.

Most of these calories should come from carbohydrate (60-70%) rich foods, which is the main source of energy. Protein (10-15%) provides with amino acids which are used by muscles to rebuild themselves. Protein intake of 1.2-2 gram/kg body weight is recommended based on specific sports activity. Fats are another source of energy and help in maintaining energy levels during exercise. Hydration is another important element in the diet. A human body is made up of up to 70 % of water and hence maintaining the right hydration level is important for its functioning.

All elements are needed to be taken in a planned manner during training/event schedule.

- A pre-workout carbohydrate fuels the training and helps in recovery, protein enhances muscle building capabilities.

- During exercise including sports drink in your diet can speed up hydration and recovery.

- Fats intake should be avoided during exercise.

- Post workout protein intake within 20mins of finishing your training is highly recommended. It helps in maintaining muscle tissues and enhances recovery and performance.

Nutrition for recovery is as much important as for training. Proper nutrition post workout boosts adaptation from the training session, repair muscle and rehydrate the body.

References

- Nutrition, entry: newworldencyclopedia.org, Retrieved 16 January, 2019

- Fitness-sports-nutrition: verywellfit.com, Retrieved 29 March, 2019

- Carbohydrates-in-sport: gisymbol.com, Retrieved 13 May, 2019

- Sports-nutrition-how-fat-provides-energy-for-exercise: verywellfit.com, Retrieved 8 January, 2019

- The-role-of-dietary-fat, excerpt: humankinetics.com, Retrieved 21 May, 2019

- Protein-and-the-athlete, fueling-your-workout, sports-and-performance, fitness: eatright.org, Retrieved 31 March, 2019

2
Exercise and Nutrition

Exercise and nutrition enhance and maintain the physical fitness and overall health of athletes. It includes the concepts of anti-oxidants, hydration, pre and post-exercise nutrition, etc. This chapter has been carefully written to provide an easy understanding of these concepts under exercise and nutrition.

Pre-exercise Nutrition

Optimal endurance performance requires careful consideration of nutrient intake. Research accumulated over the last half-century has shown that the most beneficial nutritional intervention is one that can augment and preserve carbohydrate (CHO) fuel stores (muscle and liver glycogen) for late-race, high-intensity exercise. Consuming a meal in the hours preceding an event is one method for maximizing glycogen stores and potentially influencing its utilization during exercise.

Carbohydrate-rich Meals

Pre-exercise CHO ingestion has been a topic of controversy in recent years, likely stemming from its well-known metabolic effects. Consumption of CHO leads to a substantial increase in plasma glucose. As a result, insulin is released from the pancreas, and hepatic glucose output is blunted. Insulin initiates a signaling pathway in muscle, resulting in GLUT4 translocation and glucose uptake into the muscle cell. Increased glucose availability within muscle stimulates glycolysis and glucose oxidation. Simultaneously, insulin reduces fat oxidation. This shift in substrate utilization seems to be primarily explained by insulin-mediated inhibition of lipolysis, which reduces free fatty acid (FFA) availability. However, increased glucose uptake and oxidation reduces fat oxidation even in the presence of high intracellular concentrations of FFA, possibly as a result of reduced FFA transport into the mitochondria.

When CHO ingestion precedes exercise (up to 6 h prior), hyperinsulinemia, in combination with enhanced exercise-induced GLUT4 translocation, serves to reduce blood glucose concentrations, potentially causing early-exercise hypoglycemia in some individuals. Additionally, some, but not all, data indicate increased glycogenolysis, likely as a result of insulin-modulated FFA oxidation during exercise. These combined effects suggest a resultant reduced CHO availability late in exercise that could potentiate the early onset of fatigue. However, most studies show either no negative effects or enhanced performance with pre-exercise CHO ingestion.

Carbohydrate Feedings and Performance

In general, ingesting CHO prior to exercise appears to be beneficial to performance.

Any performance benefit derived from consuming CHO prior to exercise is likely a result of increased glycogen storage. During an overnight fast, liver glycogen stores are reduced substantially, with some studies reporting glycogenolysis rates of ~0.2–0.3 mmol glucosyl units per min during the fast, which equates to an approximate 80% reduction in liver glycogen stores overnight. Thus, sub-optimal CHO stores are likely to be present when beginning to exercise in the fasted state. Consumption of CHO prior to exercise can maximize glycogen storage. Indeed, with the use of nuclear magnetic resonance (NMR) spectroscopy, Taylor *et al.* reported that following the consumption of a mixed meal, ~20% of ingested CHO is directly stored as liver glycogen. Moreover, Coyle and colleagues reported a 42% increase in muscle glycogen storage following pre-exercise ingestion of CHO. Therefore, consuming CHO may help to increase CHO availability by maximizing CHO fuel stores prior to exercise. As such, benefits to performance may be more apparent in long-duration (>2 h) performance trials, which are likely limited by initial glycogen content. Indeed, many studies report pre-exercise CHO-mediated enhanced performance in long-duration TTE trials or pre-loaded TT. Alternatively, in studies utilizing performance trials <2 h, many studies report no change, and relatively few report enhanced performance. Worth noting, enhanced performance in shorter trials could be explained by non-metabolic, centrally-mediated effects on motor output stemming from the stimulation of CHO receptors in the mouth.

Effects of Timing

The timing of CHO intake influences its metabolic effects. Indeed, insulin and blood glucose elevations are positively correlated with CHO meal proximity to exercise. Studies in which CHO is consumed 1–4 h prior to exercise often report glucose and insulin levels declining to near-basal levels prior to exercise. Alternatively, when subjects consume CHO ≤60 min before exercise, insulin and blood glucose levels are reported to be elevated immediately prior to exercise. Interestingly, regardless of the timing of ingestion and the degree of blood glucose or insulin elevation prior to exercise, the metabolic perturbations associated with CHO meal ingestion result in an initial drop in blood glucose at the start of exercise. Although this initial drop is transient and blood glucose levels typically increase to basal levels within ~20 min, it is worth noting that the degree to which blood glucose is reduced early in exercise seems to be associated with meal proximity, with meals ingested ≤60 min pre-exercise resulting in a greater reduction.

The effect of the timing of pre-exercise CHO ingestion on performance is less clear. Studies investigating the consumption of CHO at various time points within 75 min of exercise have reported no influence of timing on performance. However, no studies have compared the effects of ingesting CHO within the hour before exercise *versus* 2–3 h prior to exercise. Of interest, in studies where subjects consumed a CHO meal 2–3 h prior to exercise, TTE and TT performance were consistently improved. Alternatively, studies comparing CHO ingestion to placebo ≤60 min prior to exercise have reported far less consistent effects on performance. With this in mind, it seems reasonable that the metabolic perturbations associated with consuming CHO within 1 h prior to exercise (*i.e.*, a large increase in blood glucose and insulin followed by a dramatic drop in blood glucose), although seemingly inconsequential when compared to placebo, may potentially impair performance when compared to CHO ingestion 2–3 h prior. Thus, it may be prudent for those susceptible to hypoglycemia to schedule their pre-race meal 2–3 h prior. Alternatively, one might consider consuming CHO during warm-up, as this has been reported to blunt pre-race glucose and insulin spikes, likely as a result of catecholamine-induced insulin inhibition.

Effects of Glycemic Index

The glycemic index (GI) refers to the degree to which a CHO elevates blood glucose in the 2 h following consumption. The higher the GI of a CHO, the more rapid is the increase in blood glucose. As such, consuming a low- *versus* high-GI CHO prior to exercise results in an attenuated blood glucose and insulin response, which may help to enhance fat oxidation and maintain euglycemia during exercise, although not all studies support this. This potentially enhanced fat oxidation may be the reason why some have noted a trend for muscle glycogen sparing with low- *versus* high-GI CHO. Alternatively, high-GI CHO, may increase glycogenolysis. With this in mind, it seems logical that the beneficial metabolic effects from consuming a low-GI CHO would benefit performance *versus* high-GI CHO via preservation of endogenous glycogen stores. However, findings have been inconsistent, with some reporting enhanced TTE and TT performance with low-GI CHO and others reporting no differences *versus* high GI CHO. These inconsistencies may be due to methodological differences (e.g., timing, amount of CHO, exercise protocol). Of note, no studies report a performance decrement resulting from low-GI CHO consumption *versus* high-GI CHO. As such, low-GI CHO represents an intriguing pre-exercise nutritional option that may benefit performance to a greater extent or, at least, equally to high-GI CHO. More research is warranted to determine the true effects of low-GI CHO, as the confirmation of its potential superiority over high-GI CHO would be quite relevant to athletes.

Multiple Transportable Carbohydrates

Besides the glycemic effects of pre-exercise CHO, other important considerations mediated by CHO type include gastric emptying, fluid delivery, absorption rates and the effects on gastrointestinal comfort. Generally, gastric emptying and fluid delivery are negatively correlated with the energy content of CHO being ingested. Absorption is a function of both gastric emptying and intestinal transporter number and activity. Gastrointestinal distress may result from malabsorption of ingested CHO. All of these variables can significantly influence the rate of CHO availability for glycogen synthesis prior to exercising, as well as the incidence of gastrointestinal distress during exercise itself.

Recent research indicates that the type and composition of CHO can influence gastric emptying, fluid delivery, absorption and gastrointestinal distress. For example, studies examining the effects of consuming glucose/maltodextrin + fructose (GF) during exercise have reported enhanced gastric emptying, fluid delivery and absorption rates *versus* isocaloric amounts of glucose alone. Moreover, consuming GF during exercise seems to attenuate gastrointestinal distress when compared to isocaloric glucose alone. These effects may be due to non-competitive CHO intestinal transport, as glucose and maltodextrin are transported into the blood stream via the sodium-dependent SGLT1 transporter and fructose via GLUT5. This "multiple transport" of CHO seems to enhance the delivery of CHO to muscle. Indeed, research has indicated that the oxidation of exogenous CHO during exercise is significantly higher with GF (1.75 g/min) *versus* isocaloric glucose alone (~1.0 g/min). This may explain the reported performance improvements with during-exercise GF *versus* isocaloric glucose alone.

While the ingestion of multiple transportable CHO (MTC) during exercise has been thoroughly researched, the effects of MTC ingestion pre-exercise have not been investigated. Presumably, due to enhanced gastric emptying, fluid delivery and CHO absorption, MTC could provide a more effective means of hydrating and increasing CHO availability prior to exercise. Furthermore, although purely speculative, if an athlete is limited to or prefers to consume additional CHO ≤1 h prior to exercising, the enhanced digestion of MTC *versus* glucose alone may help to improve gut comfort during exercise.

Modified and Resistant Starches

Interestingly, technological advances have allowed for the modification of starches via various means (e.g., hydrothermally modified starch, acid/alcohol-modified cornstarches, chemical modified starches) and represents a novel method to potentially enhance CHO availability during exercise, the importance of CHO availability to exercise performance is well-established, and it can be accomplished in one of three ways: (1) providing exogenous CHO to serve as a fuel source; (2) altering substrate utilization in a way that preserves endogenous CHO; or (3) a combination of the two. Traditionally, starches can be classified as either slowly or rapidly digestible based on their rate of glucose release and their absorption rate upon ingestion. More specifically, the varying rates of digestibility are traditionally dependent upon the amylose:amylopectin ratio of their structural makeup, with a higher ratio increasing the resistance to digestion. However, by modifying starches, the gastric-emptying rate can be manipulated despite the amylose:amylopectin ratio. Thus, these modification techniques can either enhance or inhibit the glycemic and insulinemic responses. Logically, this could enhance glycogen storage pre- or post-exercise or spare glycogen during exercise by enhancing fat oxidation.

While there is some evidence of beneficial metabolic effects from consuming modified starches in certain clinical populations (e.g., diabetics), data on the performance effects is limited. Moreover, because the type of modification results in either a slow- or fast-digesting starch, it is important to view the limited data based upon the digestion rate. As such, fast-digesting modified starches, such as Vitargo, may benefit performance. Stephens *et al.* examined the implications of consuming a high molecular weight (HMW) rapidly-digested modified starch (Vitargo), a low molecular weight (LMW) glucose polymer derived from hydrolyzed corn starch representing a maltodextrin recovery drink or sugar-free water on muscle glycogen resynthesis and endurance performance. Following a glycogen-depleting, submaximal cycling test (75% of maximal oxygen uptake (VO_{2max}), subjects consumed one of the aforementioned drinks and then rested for 2 h. Immediately after the 2-h rest, those who consumed the HMW or LMW starch exhibited a significantly greater work output on a 15-min all-out cycling test in comparison to the sugar-free water group ($p < 0.001$ and $p < 0.01$, respectively). In addition, the HMW group had a 10% increase in work output in comparison to the LMW group ($p < 0.01$). Thus, this fast-digesting modified starch seems beneficial when consumed between exercise bouts; however, its effects on performance when consumed <2 h pre-exercise has not been investigated.

High-fat Meals

With the importance of endogenous CHO stores on endurance performance well established, recent studies have begun to examine various nutritional and training methods with the aim of optimizing performance through the manipulation of substrate utilization during exercise. The prevailing concept behind the majority of this research is to use macronutrient manipulation to determine the correct interplay between maximizing endogenous CHO storage and optimizing the capacity for fat oxidation to ultimately improve endurance performance. Due to the fact that endurance training has been shown to increase the metabolic capacity to oxidize fat during submaximal exercise, it seems logical that increasing the ability of endurance athletes to utilize an alternative fuel source to CHO (*i.e.*, fat) would improve endurance performance.

Consumption of a high-fat meal pre-exercise alters substrate supply before exercise and leads to increased free fatty acid (FFA) levels in the blood. Increased FFA levels will increase lipid metabolism during exercise and either preserve endogenous CHO stores or attenuate the normal rate of CHO depletion. While studies have shown significant performance enhancement as a result of increasing fat availability (via diet) in animals or in humans with heparin administration, the effects of consuming a high fat meal on subsequent exercise performance are equivocal.

Acute High-dat Ingestion and Performance

In contrast to a "fat adaptation" approach over a period of days or weeks, another method to improve performance is to increase fat availability acutely through the consumption of a high-fat meal within the hours (≤4 h) prior to exercise. While chronic (≥1 week) consumption of a high-fat, low-CHO diet impairs endurance performance as a result of decreasing endogenous CHO stores, consuming a single high-fat meal prior to exercise theoretically would allow for both maximal endogenous CHO storage as a result of traditional CHO-loading in the days prior to the event, as well as immediate fatty acid availability from the pre-exercise meal. However, despite these metabolic benefits, most studies report no performance benefits from consuming a pre-exercise high-fat meal when compared to a high-CHO meal.

Interestingly, Murakami et al. recently examined the performance effect of consuming either: (1) a high-fat meal 4 h pre-exercise + a placebo jelly 3 min before exercise (HFM + P); (2) a high-fat meal 4 h pre-exercise + maltodextrin jelly 3 min before exercise (HFM + M); or (3) a high-CHO meal 4 h pre-exercise + placebo jelly 3 min before exercise (HCM + P); after consuming an isocaloric, high-CHO diet for three days (2562 ± 19 kcal). Meals consumed 4 h pre-exercise were isocaloric (1007 ± 21 kcal); however, maltodextrin added 410 ± 8 kcal, while the placebo added 0 kcal. This tested eight collegiate male distance runners (mean VO_{2max} of 61.3 ± 2.2 mL/ kg/min) for an 80 min submaximal run on a treadmill at each runner's pre-determined lactate threshold (LT) speed, immediately followed by a time trial to exhaustion (TTE). Participants in the HFM + M group exhibited both a significantly higher fat oxidation rate and a significantly decreased CHO oxidation rate during the first 60 min of exercise compared to the HCM + P group. This suggests that CHO feeding subsequent to a HFM pre-exercise and three days of a proper CHO loading protocol can elicit an enhancement in the endurance performance of well-trained runners. The increased fat oxidation and decreased CHO oxidation during the first 60 min of exercise theoretically leads to an increase in glycogen stores at the end of exercise, thus improving TTE performance. Worth noting, a significant increase in TTE duration in the HFM + M group (100 ± 3.4 min) compared to the HFM + P (92 ± 2.8 min) or HCM + P groups (90 ± 1.7 min) was reported; however, Murakami and colleagues did not include a HCM + M group, which raises questions about whether the HFM + M group performed longer primarily due to HFM or rather as a result of the increased caloric consumption of maltodextrin immediately pre-exercise.

Furthermore, these findings are in direct contrast to others comparing pre-exercise high-CHO meal consumption to high fat and should be interpreted with caution, due to methodological considerations.

Worth noting, another potential factor that may need to be addressed is the fact that the majority of research methodology pertaining to acute pre-exercise fat feeding has used cycling as the exercise modality. The work of Murakami *et al.* prompts the questioning of the importance of the exercise modality in eliciting significant changes. Though strictly theoretical, perhaps the muscle recruitment mechanics of the individual exercise modalities differentially influences the metabolic effects resulting from various pre-exercise macronutrient manipulations.

Mixed CHO-protein Meals

Much research has been done in recent years investigating the effects of adding protein (PRO) to CHO (CHO-PRO) beverages or supplements during exercise and post-exercise. Findings have been intriguing with some, but not others, reporting enhanced TTE and TT performance with during-exercise CHO-PRO *versus* CHO intake alone. Additionally, some, but not all, studies investigating the effects of post-exercise CHO-PRO intake on subsequent exercise performance have also noted enhanced TTE and TT performance, possibly as a result of increased glycogen resynthesis. Despite these findings, there has been very little research done analyzing the effects of pre-exercise CHO-PRO in the performance context. Thus, a complete understanding of CHO-PRO pre-exercise effects requires the examination of research in non-athletic populations.

Research examining the clinical implications of CHO-PRO consumption prior to exercise has helped to elucidate its metabolic effects. Adding PRO to CHO seems to attenuate the glycemic response compared to CHO alone. These effects may be partly explained by PRO-induced hormonal alterations, which are attributed to elevated levels of certain amino acids in the blood. Specifically, elevations in arginine, leucine and phenylalanine stimulate both β and α cells of the pancreas, resulting in the secretion of both insulin and glucagon, respectively. While the PRO-induced glucagon reaction is completely unique from CHO intake, the post-feeding insulin rise is also distinctively high with CHO-PRO *versus* CHO, because insulin seems to respond additively to glucose and amino acid elevations. The combined effects of these hormonal increases may, via insulin, enhance glucose disposal and, simultaneously, via glucagon, stimulate hepatic glucose output, thereby helping to maintain euglycemia. It is also worth noting that due to higher insulin levels with CHO-PRO, FFA oxidation may be reduced to a greater degree *versus* CHO. However, this effect may be partially counterbalanced by the potentially lipolytic effects of glucagon.

Besides the potential protection from early-exercise hypoglycemia, CHO-PRO ingestion may also enhance pre-exercise fuel storage. Several mechanistic studies in rodents have determined that pre-exercise PRO consumption can enhance glycogen synthesis and may lead to glycogen sparing during exercise. With this evidence in rodents in combination with the evidence of enhanced post-exercise glycogen resynthesis, it seems plausible that pre-exercise CHO-PRO ingestion could augment glycogen storage pre-exercise in humans. However, while it is tempting to speculate that CHO-PRO ingestion prior to exercise could enhance exercise capacity or performance in humans by augmenting and sparing glycogen stores, there is little evidence to support or refute this notion.

Protein Feedings and Performance

There is only one study analyzing the effects of a PRO meal on subsequent endurance exercise metabolism and performance. Using trained cyclists, Rowlands and Hopkins investigated the effects of the pre-exercise (90 min) ingestion of three different fuels ((1) CHO; (2) PRO; or (3) a high-fat meal) on late-exercise TT and sprint performance (following ~2 h of cycling). Specifically, the CHO meal increased insulin and decreased FFA oxidation levels to a greater degree than fat or PRO. These findings are somewhat unexpected based on reports of higher insulin levels and lower FFA oxidation with CHO-PRO intake *versus* CHO alone. However, , soy protein was utilized, which may have influenced the insulinemic response differently from other types of protein (e.g., whey) . Perhaps the use of whey PRO would have resulted in a greater insulin response, potentially enhancing glycogen storage and during-exercise metabolism, although this idea is purely speculative. Further worth noting, subjects consumed a CHO drink during exercise. The maintenance of plasma glucose levels in all trials may have blunted the effects of a PRO meal, which may explain why no performance differences were observed. Furthermore, the long trial duration (3+ h) may have influenced reliability (3.7% within-subject error for 50 km TT), making it more difficult to detect statistical differences. Therefore, more research is necessary to determine the true effects of pre-exercise CHO-PRO consumption.

Nutrition while Exercising

It is very important to make sure where appropriate, that food and fluid is ingested during exercise, in both training and competition.

During moderate to high intensity exercise the body uses predominantly carbohydrate as a fuel source, as well as some fat storage. Carbohydrate fuel comes in the form of muscle glycogen and blood glucose. Depending on many factors, many sports can adequately be completed with focus on nutritional preparation. Our carbohydrate (and fat) storage covers most fuel needs, if well prepared. Fluid however is vital for during exercise for majority of activities, as sweat rate begins so does the bodies need for fuel intake.

Food

Consuming food during exercise has the number one aim to improve performance in a competition, and also to lift work rate, or the ability to do the given work load during a training session.

Benefits of Intake

Specific benefits of consuming carbohydrate during exercise are to firstly keep blood glucose levels high during prolonged moderate-high intensity events. Blood glucose provides an alternative fuel source for the muscle when glycogen storage levels are getting low. Carbohydrate during exercise also provides a fuel source for the brain to maintain skills and decision making, and reduce the perception of fatigue. Lastly, intake of glucose can spare or replenishing muscle glycogen. It is believed that during low intensity work, carbohydrate consumed during exercise can be burned to save glycogen stores or can replenish glycogen stores for use later.

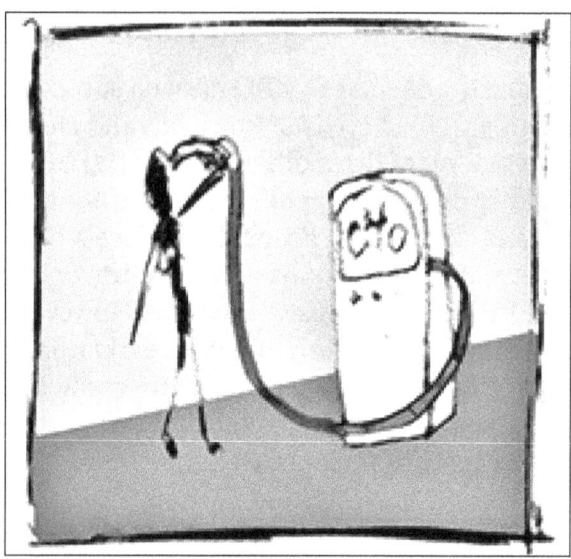

Identifying factors that determine the appropriateness of consumption during exercise, is crucial in deciding if carbohydrate is needed for you.

- Generally, the longer the event, the greater the amount of carbohydrate that is utilized. As a rule of thumb, if your sport or training is longer than an hour, you may benefit from consuming some carbohydrates during sport in addition to fluid.

- Higher intensity exercise will burn more glycogen, or fuels stores more quickly during your game or session. So if your exercise session is roughly an hour and consists of predominantly high intensity work, then taking in some carbohydrate may be beneficial.

- Temperature will also play a role, in that the hotter it is, the quicker glycogen will be used. However, in these situations, it is more likely that overheating and dehydration will be the limitation to performance.

- Pre-exercise eating has an impact on glycogen storage. The better ones pre-exercise meal is, the higher the stores of carbohydrate will be, and hence the more fuel that will be available for conversion during that event or session.

Food intake during exercise should be easy to swallow with limited chewing. Liquid options are often the best options, however this will depend on personal preference and ability to stomach certain foods. Each of the following options provides about 50g carbohydrate:

- 800 ml sports drink.

- 500 ml cola drink.

- Liquid meal supplement.

- 1 sports bars.

- 2 sports gels.

- 3 small or 2 large bananas.

Post-exercise Nutrition

A post-exercise meal aids in replenishing the energy you've used up during your workout. It also improves the size and quality of your muscles and repairs the damage you've caused during the activity. Beyond simply repairing the body from the workout, it also helps provide nutrition and hydration.

The importance of recovery nutrition depends on the type and duration of exercise just completed, body composition goals and personal preferences. The goals of the recovery nutrition are to:

- Appropriately refuel and rehydrate the body.

- Promote muscle repair and growth.

- Boost adaptation from the training session.

- Support immune function.

Proactive recovery nutrition is especially important if you complete two or more training sessions in one day or two sessions in close succession (e.g. evening session followed by early morning session the next day). However, if you're exercising once a day or a couple of times a week, recovery nutrition is still important but you may be able to meet your nutrition goals from your usual meals or snacks than adding in extra food.

Consequences of Inadequate Nutrition

Inadequate nutrition recovery, especially if training multiple times a day, can result in:

- Increased fatigue (during training and at work or school).

- Reduced performance at your next training session or event.

- Suboptimal gains from the session just completed.

- Increased muscle soreness.

Recovery Nutrition Timing

Rehydrating should begin soon after finishing your training session or event, however, the urgency for carbohydrate and protein after exercise depends on how long you have until your next exercise session. The body is most effective at replacing carbohydrate and promoting muscle repair and growth in the first ~60-90 min after exercise, however this will continue to occur for another ~12-24 hr. So, if you have a quick turn around between sessions it's a good idea to maximise your recovery in the first 60-90 minutes after you finish exercising. Otherwise you could use your next regular meal after the session as your recovery nutrition. Some people may benefit from splitting their recovery into two parts with a small snack soon after exercise to kick start the recovery process followed by their next main meal to complete their recovery goals.

Recovery Food Guide

Everyone is different in what they like to eat, what their appetite is like and what sits comfortably in their stomach in the hours after exercise but in general foods should:

- Be rich in quality carbohydrate to replenish muscle fuel stores.

- Contain some lean protein to promote muscle repair.

- Include a source of fluid and electrolytes to rehydrate effectively.

There's no one "best" option for what to eat after exercise. Dairy foods such as flavoured milk, smoothies or fruit yoghurt can be a great option as they can provide carbohydrate, protein, fluid and electrolytes ticking all of your recovery goals in one handy option. Some other options that you may like to choose include:

- Lean chicken and salad roll.

- Bowl of muesli with yoghurt and berries.

- Fresh fruit salad topped with Greek yoghurt.

- Spaghetti with lean beef bolognaise sauce.

- Chicken burrito with salad and cheese.

- Small tin of tuna on crackers plus a banana.

Best Fluid to Drink Post-exercise

The ideal fluid during exercise depends on your goals. If you are using fluid mainly to rehydrate from the session than water or electrolyte drinks are a good option. If you are also drinking to meet your source of carbohydrate goals then sports drinks can be helpful as they contain both carbohydrates and fluid to help hydrate and fuel your body at the same time. Dairy based fluids such as smoothies and flavoured milk are especially handy if you want to protein, carbohydrate, fluid and electrolyte in one go. Specialised protein powders and recovery shakes may be useful in some situations for some people however, for many people their recovery goals can be met using regular foods and drinks.

Anti-oxidants

While oxygen is vital for life of an aerobic organism, the by-products of its metabolism can be harmful to cells. The very small not-to-water-reduced part of oxygen leads to the production of reactive oxygen intermediates, also known as ROS. This is happening ubiquitary but in particular in the working muscle during or after exercise. ROS includes superoxide ($O_2^{\cdot-}$), nitric oxide ($NO^{\cdot}$) and hydroxyl radicals ($HO^{\cdot}$) and also non-radicals such as singlet oxygen ($^{1}O_2$) or hydrogen peroxide (H_2O_2). Depending on the type of exercise, a number of potential mechanisms for the generation of ROS within the muscle have been proposed, such as: (a) increased formation of $O_2^{\cdot-}$ in the mitochondrial respiratory chain, (b) xanthine oxidase (XO) catalysed degradation of AMP (adenosine monophosphate) during ischaemic muscular work leading to increased production of O_2^{-}, (c) increased ROS formation in the oxidative-burst reaction due to activation of polymorphoneutrophils (PMNs) after exercise-induced muscle damage, (d) loss of calcium homeostasis in stressed muscles, (e) enhanced cytokine production and activation of nuclear factor kappa B (NF-κB), catecholamine autooxidation and many more. Owing to the unpaired electron in its outer orbit, ROS tend to extract electrons from other molecules to reach a chemically more stable state. However, the generation of ROS is per se not harmful and necessary for the proper functioning of metabolic processes, muscular contraction and immune defence. Muscle antioxidant defence systems are upregulated in response to exercise. NF-κB and mitogen-activated protein kinase are the two major oxidative-stress-sensitive signal transduction pathways that have been shown to activate the gene expression of a number of enzymes and proteins that play important roles in maintenance of intracellular oxidant–antioxidant homeostasis.

It is only when the body's natural antioxidant defence system is insufficient to detoxify formed ROS that oxidative stress with damage or destruction of cellular macromolecules such as lipids, proteins, nucleic acids and components of the extracellular matrix may occur. Oxidative stress has been associated with decreased physical performance, muscular fatigue, muscle damage and overtraining. Therefore, it is sometimes suggested that reducing oxidative stress (e.g. by antioxidant supplementation) would improve exercise tolerance and performance. However, to minimise oxidative stress, the organism contains a powerful antioxidant defence system that depends on nutritionally derived antioxidant vitamins such as vitamin E and C, β-carotene, flavonoids, polyphenols as well as endogenous antioxidant (enzyme) compounds, such as glutathione (GSH), catalase (CAT) and superoxide dismutase (SOD). Therefore, oxidative stress during or following exercise can occur only if the exercise-induced generation of ROS is higher than the detoxifying potential of the antioxidant defence systems. Many studies have investigated the effect of physical exercise with respect to the onset and magnitude of oxidative stress and the protective role of antioxidants, however, with various outcomes. There is strong support for the assumption that the manifold designs and methods employed to induce and measure oxidative stress are a major cause for conflicting results: Factors such as gender, age, type of exercise (concentric vs. eccentric, maximal vs. submaximal etc.), level and years of training and particularly the exercise-induced local and systemic stress response could account for both differences in ROS generation and the development of antioxidant defence mechanisms. Nevertheless, antioxidants, either endogenously produced or dietary substances that can act as antioxidants, play a major role in the whole network.

Antioxidant Defence Mechanisms

The protective mechanisms against oxidative stress can be divided into two major categories: endogenously produced enzymatic antioxidants that include SOD, glutathione peroxidase (GPX), CAT, glutaredoxin (GRX) and thioredoxin (TRX). Non-enzymatic antioxidants include nutritionally derived vitamins and provitamins (vitamin E, vitamin C and β-carotene), flavonoids and polyphenols, proteins such as thiols (mainly GSH) and various other low-molecular-weight compounds as ubiquinone, uric acid (UA) and many more. These substances can either prevent ROS formation or scavenge radical species and convert them into a less active molecule. Furthermore, they avoid the transformation of less active ROS (e.g. O_2^{-}) into more potent forms (e.g. HO·), enhance the resistance of sensitive biological targets to ROS attack and assist in the repair of radical-induced damage. Although most antioxidants are located in specific cellular sites or compartments, they act synergistically and some of them cooperate in the so-called antioxidant chain reaction. This means that, for example, the –SH pool from reduced GSH regenerates vitamins C and E and vitamin C recycles vitamin E. In contrast to other vertebrates, the human organism is not able to synthesise antioxidant vitamins; therefore, non-enzymatic antioxidants such as vitamin E, vitamin C, β-carotene, polyphenols and flavonoids have to be provided by the diet. This implies that the plasma and tissue levels of these non-enzymatic antioxidants are dependent on the quality of foods. In contrast, the enzymatic antioxidants are synthesised within the human organism and several lines of evidence suggest that their production can be upregulated in response to chronic exposure to oxidants. Although the response may depend on exercise intensity or training duration, most studies have reported an increase in antioxidant enzyme activity following chronic physical exercise. This may represent an important mechanism to explain findings from some investigations showing less oxidative stress in trained individuals.

Table: Enzymatic and non-enzymatic anti-oxidants, locations and main functions.

Enzymatic Antioxidants	Location	Function
SOD	Mitochondria, cytosol	Dismutates superoxide radicals
GPX	Mitochondria, cytosol and cell membrane	Reduces hydrogen peroxide and organic hydroperoxides
CAT	Peroxisomes	Reduces hydrogen peroxide
GRX	Cytosol	Protects and repairs protein and non-protein thiols
TRX	Cytosol	Catalyses the reduction of protein S–S bridges
		Removes hydrogen peroxide
		Scavenges free radicals
Non-enzymatic Antioxidants	Location	Function
Vitamin C	Aqueous phase of cells	Scavenges free radicals
		Recycles vitamin E
Vitamin E, mainly α- and γ-tocopherol	Cell membranesa	Breaks lipid peroxidation chain reactions, reduces several ROS to less reactive forms
Carotenoids	Cell membranesa	Scavenges free radicals
		Protects against lipid peroxidation
Glutathion	Ubiquitary non-protein thiol	Scavenges free radicals
		Removes hydrogen and organic peroxides in a GPX-catalysed reaction
		Recycles various antioxidants (vitamin C, E)
Flavonoids/polyphenols	Cell membranesa	Scavenges free radicals
		Metal chelator
Ubiquinones	Cell membranesa	Scavenges oxygen radicals and singlet oxygen
		Recycles vitamin E
UA	Ubiquitary	Scavenges HO radicals

Antioxidant Supplementation and Exercise-induced Oxidative Stress

Over the past few decades, there have been plenty of exercise studies with measures of oxidative stress as the main outcome when using antioxidant supplementations.

The most common antioxidants used were vitamin E and vitamin C and various antioxidant combinations, also including the latter vitamins. More recently, polyphenols or supplements containing them have been investigated. Not very often, carotenoids, selenium α-lipoic acid or *N*-acetylcysteine have been used. To draw a general conclusion, it can be said that the outcome was inconsistent, from lowering a oxidative stress biomarker to also increasing then.

Furthermore, on the population level, many studies have revealed that the 'classical' antioxidants C and E are not only effective in reducing the risk of chronic diseases, but also increasing them slightly.

Antioxidants and their Action

Since it is a common practice for athletes to use antioxidants, there is a wide range of vitamins, minerals and different extracts marketed as supplements. However, very often, not in the most active form, overdosed when compared to recommended daily allowances (RDIs), not highly bioavailable and especially as an extract, not even well characterised. Many of the orally taken supplements also have an impact on the antioxidative enzymes or GSH.

Glutathione

GSH is the most abundant non-protein thiol source in the muscle. Its concentration in the cells is usually in a millimolar range but is having a wide range across organs depending on their radical production. It serves various roles in the cellular defence system by directly scavenging radicals, removing hydrogen and organic peroxides, recycling a variety of other antioxidants such as vitamin E and reducing semi-dehydroascorbate radicals. The various ways of acting and the interaction with exogenic substances show the dependency of the GSH activity on the consumption of substances acting as antioxidants.

The same is true for SOD, CAT or glutathionperoxidase, which belongs to the consumption of their active micronutrients such as iron, manganese, zinc or selenium.

Bilirubin and UA

Bilirubin and UA represent important endogenous antioxidants mainly found in the plasma. UA serves as a free radical scavenger, can trap peroxyl radicals in aqueous phases and therefore contribute to the plasma antioxidant defence. During exercise, energy-rich purine phosphates are used and catabolised, resulting in accumulation of hypoxanthine, xanthine and UA in tissues. The conversion of hypoxanthine into xanthine and UA is associated with the formation of toxic oxygen-free radicals.

Plasma concentrations of the potent hydrophilic antioxidant UA are known to increase during intense exercise, produced from increased purine metabolism and probably also because of impaired renal clearance.

Bilirubin has been shown to efficiently scavenge peroxyl radicals and act as a metal-binding species, thus functioning as a selective antioxidant. Similar to UA, bilirubin has also been shown to increase after exercise. Since bilirubin is released into the plasma fluid by destruction of red blood cells, haemolysis which arises during physical activity (e.g. during marathon distance running) can be one explanation.

However, there is now novel information published on hyperbilirubinaemia, showing significant antioxidative effects, protection from non-communicable diseases (NCDs) such as cardiovascular disease (CVD) and cancer as well as a severe impact on lipid metabolism. Released bilirubin in the plasma is immediately bound to albumin in blood and transported to the liver. In the liver, unconjugated bilirubin is conjugated to glucuronic acid, consequently gets water soluble and is finally called conjugated bilirubin. A mutation in the gene promoter region of bilirubinuridine–diphosphate–glucuronyl transferase (40–60% impaired glucuronidation) can cause hyperbilirubinaemia, arising in approximately 5–10% of the general population. So far, no link has been drawn to physical activity and adaptation processes in hyperbilirubinaemic subjects, but it is highly expected that a high bilirubin plasma concentration has significant effects on metabolism during physical activity.

Vitamin E: A Group of Tocopherols

Very often, it is ignored that the term vitamin E represents a family of eight natural, structurally related compounds. These compounds contain a chromanol ring with a phytyl side chain, which is saturated for tocopherols and unsaturated for tocotrienols. The α-, β-, γ- and δ-tocopherols and the α-, β-, γ- and δ-tocotrienols differ in the number and the position of methyl groups substituted on the ring.

The forms of vitamin E in most supplements are the synthetic all-rac-α-tocopheryl acetate or all-rac-α-tocopheryl succinate; however, both show not the highest vitamin E activity.

Of all compounds with vitamin E activity, α- and γ-tocopherols are the principal vitamins found in human and animal diets and comprise most of the vitamin E content of tissues.

Interestingly, the intake of γ-tocopherol has been estimated to exceed that of α-tocopherol by a factor of 2–4 in North America. This is due to the fact that soya bean oil is the predominant vegetable oil in the American diet (76.4%) followed by corn oil and canola oil (both 7%). In Europe, the consumption of the α-form exceeds γ-tocopherol with a ratio of approximately 2:1. However, most of the supplementation studies in exercise science and also on the population level to prevent chronic diseases have been performed with α-tocopherol.

The ability to donate the phenolic hydrogen is thus very important for the antioxidant activity of the tocopherols as they scavenge the peroxyl radicals. The lack of the C-5 methyl group decreases the electron density in the phenolic ring, making γ-tocopherol a less potent hydrogen donor than α-tocopherol. The bond dissociation energies for the phenolic hydrogens are 75.8 and 79.6 Kcal/mole in the case of α- and γ-tocopherols, respectively. This makes α-tocopherol a more efficient hydrogen donor and radical scavenger than γ-tocopherol. However, the higher hydrogen-donation ability is a double-edged sword as it makes α-tocopherol participate more readily in side reactions, leading to partial loss of its antioxidant activity. This also contributes to the negative findings of high dose supplementation with various α-tocopherol forms.

Vitamin C

In contrast to tocopherols is vitamin C (ascorbic acid) hydrophilic which acts better in the aqueous environment. It is widely distributed but found in high amounts in leukocytes, adrenal and pituitary glands. Besides its scavenging activity, it is well known to recycle the tocopherol radical, thereby being reduced to the dehydroascorbic acid which can then be regenerated, for example, by GSH.

Some decades ago, the intake of vitamin C was too low; however, nowadays, owing to the availability of fruits and vegetables, the intake has increased and vitamin C is enriched in almost every food, particularly meat and sausages, as antioxidant. Therefore, the vitamin C intake via dietary sources exceeds the recommendations nowadays.

Further, pharmacokinetic data indicate a plasma steady state after a vitamin C intake of 200 mg, whereas the ascorbic acid contents of neutrophils, monocytes and lymphocytes are saturated at a daily intake of 100 mg. Similar to α-tocopherol, it is also well known that vitamin C turns its antioxidative activity towards pro-oxidative activity after high dose supplementation, particularly in the presence of transition metals such as Fe^{3+}.

Taking the latter into consideration, the total intake of vitamin C should not exceed the recommendations manifold. Furthermore, recent studies have shown that antioxidative supplements (mainly vitamins C and E) hinder the beneficial cell adaptation to exercise.

β-carotene

Supplementation with carotenoids, particularly β-carotene, should be done with care and with hands on the dose. Particularly for β-carotene, no acceptable daily intake (ADI) is set, since it contributes to an increased risk of cancer (particularly lung cancer) in heavy smokers at an intake of 20 mg/day or higher. Carotenoids act along two different main pathways—physical and chemical radical quenching. Physical quenching implies the deactivation of singlet oxygen by energy transfer to the excited oxygen species leading to the carotenoid, yielding a triplet-exciting carotenoid. The energy of this carotenoid is dissipated to recover the ground state; the carotenoid itself remains interactive in the process and is able to undergo more cycles of deactivation. Chemical quenching contributes <0.05% to the total $^1O_2$-quenching by carotenoids, but is responsible for the eventual destruction of the molecule. Besides this quenching ability, carotenoids are able to scavenge peroxyl radicals by chemical interactions. However, mainly, β-carotene acts only at low oxygen partial pressure as antioxidant; hyperoxide conditions, often present during and after physical activity, results in a shift to a pro-oxidant.

Further Antioxidants in Use

Flavonoids are a family of secondary active plant constituents which have been associated with antioxidative potential, although very often only in in vitro studies. The most prominent ones are flavonones, isoflavonones, flavanones, anthocyanins and catechins. Their biological activities are very broad such as anti-inflammatory, anti-mutagen, anti-tumoral or anti-ischaemic. Most of the observed activities are based on their anti-oxidative potential as a radical scavenger. As polyphenols, they also act as a regenerator of vitamin E radicals or β-carotene. Since they are broadly found in plant products such as black or green tea, grapes and red wine, supplementation must be considered with care. Many of the supplements carrying 'plant extracts' are not well defined and concentrations should be carefully evaluated, if given at all. Furthermore, they could contain contaminants, which are doing more harm than good and were also responsible for ending the careers of athletes. One other crucial point is their bioavailability which is regularly very low.

However, recent studies could show the beneficial effects of polyphenols or extracts (grape, beet-root, Rhodiola rosa or Eckonia cava algae) with regard to oxidative stress in physically active persons, but no effects such as ergogenic acids. Further, they did not improve muscle force output.

Solely, the antioxidant mechanisms cannot be responsible for the observed effects of polyphenols; therefore, other links are proposed such as the influence on cell-signalling cascades and the interaction with key proteins in these cascades.

Ubiquinones are lipid-soluble quinone derivatives containing an isoprene or farnesyl tail. In humans, predominantly, ubiquinone-10, also called coenzyme-Q, is bioactive. It is found in the diet (soy bean oil, nuts, fish and meat) but also, very often, supplementation is taking place. The antioxidant effects are attributed to their phenolic ring structure, which acts as a radical scavenger, but it is also used to regenerate other primary antioxidants such as tocopherols.

Coenzyme-Q is very popular among athletes, but shows no significant benefit on exercise performance, regardless of age or training status. However, positive effects by Q_{10} were also shown, such as improved VO_{2max}, faster recovery rate and fatigue recovery.

Hydration

Water is essential to maintain blood volume, regulate body temperature and allow muscle contractions to take place. During exercise, the main way the body maintains optimal body temperature is by sweating. Heat is removed from the body when beads of sweat on the skin evaporate, resulting in a loss of body fluid. Sweat production, and therefore fluid loss, increases with a rise in ambient temperature and humidity, as well as with an increase in exercise intensity.

Drinking fluid during exercise is necessary to replace fluids lost in sweat. This action will reduce the risk of heat stress, maintain normal muscle function, and prevent performance decreases due to dehydration. In most cases during exercise, the rates of sweat loss are higher than the rate you can drink, so most athletes get into fluid deficit. Therefore, fluid guidelines promote drinking more fluid to reduce the deficit and potential performance detriments associated with dehydration. However, it is also important to acknowledge that it is possible to over-drink during exercise. This highlights the importance of getting to know your sweat rate and knowing how much you should be drinking.

Dehydration and Performance

As dehydration increases, there is a gradual reduction in physical and mental performance. There is an increase in heart rate and body temperature, and an increased perception of how hard the exercise feels, especially when exercising in the heat. Studies show that loss of fluid equal to 2% of body mass is sufficient to cause a detectable decrease in performance (that's a 1.4 kg loss in a 70 kg athlete). Dehydration of greater than 2% loss of body weight increases the risk of nausea, vomiting, diarrhoea, and other gastro-intestinal problems during exercise.

Dehydration reduces the rate of fluid absorption from the intestines, making it more difficult to reverse the fluid deficit. You may end up feeling bloated and sick if you delay fluid replacement. It is impossible to 'train' or 'toughen' your body to handle dehydration.

Drinking more fluid than is comfortable, in any conditions, has the potential to interfere with your performance. In cool weather or when the exercise pace is gentle, the rate of sweat loss may be quite low. It is unnecessary and potentially dangerous to drink at rates that are far greater than sweat losses. Such over-hydration during exercise can cause a dilution of blood sodium levels (hyponatraemia). Symptoms include headaches, disorientation, coma, and in severe cases, death. It is important to note though that this is relatively rare and dehydration is a much more common issue.

Estimating your Fluid Losses

Knowing your sweat rate can give you an indication of how much you should be drinking during exercise. Sports dietitians routinely measure an athlete's sweat rate during training and competition in a range of environmental conditions, to provide them with the information required to design an individual fluid plan. Follow these easy steps to measure your fluid losses:

- Weigh yourself in minimal clothing, as close to the start of exercise as possible. Ideally you should empty your bladder before weighing.

- Commence exercise session.

- Weigh yourself at the end of your session, in minimal clothing again, ensuring you towel off any excess sweat from your body.

- Your weight change during exercise reflects your total fluid loss; i.e. the difference between your sweat losses and fluid intake.

- Remember that weight loss during exercise is primarily water loss (not fat loss), and needs to be replaced soon after finishing exercise.

- Other minor losses come from breathing, spitting, vomiting and other insignificant sources. Sweat losses can be monitored to give you an idea of how much fluid to replace during training sessions and competition.

Fluid Quantity and Timing

Drinking fluid during exercise helps to prevent a drop in performance caused by dehydration, and fluid after exercise will re-hydrate you. The amount of fluid and the timing of drinks depend on the individual and the sport. Here are some tips:

- Always start exercise well hydrated; this will lower the risk of becoming dehydrated during sport. There is minimal performance benefit to being over-hydrated as drinking excessive amounts of fluid before exercise causes increased urination and feeling bloated.

- Develop a plan for drinking during exercise based on your own sweat rates.

- Immediately after exercise, monitor your weight change to estimate your final fluid deficit. During recovery, you will continue to lose fluids through sweating and urine losses, so plan to replace 125-150% of this fluid deficit over the next 2-6 hours. For example, if you lost 1 kg (1000mL), you will need to drink 1250-1500 mL to fully re-hydrate. Drink fluids with your recovery snacks and the following meal to achieve this goal.

- Different sports pose different challenges and opportunities for optimal hydration. For team and racquet sports there are formal breaks between play, with substitutions and time-outs, all offering an opportunity to drink. Some individual sports require you to drink on the move. Be smart and practice strategies to get maximum benefit from fluid intake with minimal fuss and discomfort. Try special squeeze bottles, or hands free drink pouches if practical.

- Thirst is not an effective indicator of hydration status while exercising. There is usually a significant fluid loss before you feel thirsty. When drinking, your thirst will be satisfied well before these losses have been fully replaced.

Best Fluid to Drink

As there are many drink options available, you now need to think about which is best for you. Plain water alone is an effective drink for fluid replacement, especially in low intensity and short duration sports. However, if carbohydrate and electrolytes are added to water, as in a sports drink, performance can be enhanced, especially in high intensity and endurance sports.

If a drink tastes good, athletes will consume more of it, which may assist in meeting fluid targets during competition or rehydrating more effectively. Carbohydrate in fluid provides a muscle energy source as well as enhancing flavour. This can be one advantage of a sports drink over plain water. Electrolytes such as sodium are lost in sweat and need to be replaced during and after prolonged exercise. Sodium in fluid improves fluid intake as it stimulates the thirst mechanism, promotes both carbohydrate and water uptake in the intestines, and reduces the volume of urine produced post-exercise. Of course, salt can be consumed in foods that are eaten at the same time as post-exercise fluids.

Caffeine

There is a growing number of drinks on the market that contain a number of ingredients including caffeine. Caffeine is no longer banned by the World Anti Doping Agency. The consumption of small to moderate doses of caffeine (75 - 200 mg) can help to sustain exercise performance, reduce the perception of effort, and is unlikely to alter hydration status during exercise. However, the use of caffeine amongst athletes is often ad hoc and they may be unaware of the potential detrimental side effects associated with its use. Ensure that you discuss the use of caffeine with your sports dietitian or sports scientist and consider individual responses to caffeine.

Alcohol

Alcohol is not a suitable fluid to choose immediately after exercise, as it will impair vital recovery processes, and may also impair the athlete's ability to rehydrate effectively. If you choose to drink alcohol after exercise, look after your recovery needs first (i.e. replacing fluids, carbohydrate stores and consuming some protein to assist with muscle repair) and then enjoy an alcoholic beverage in sensible amounts.

Common Guidelines

- The detrimental effects of dehydration on performance may include: loss of coordination, impaired ability to make a decision, increased rate of perceived exertion and increased risk of heat stress.

- Aim to match your sweat rate with fluid intake as closely as possible.

- Ensure that you drink at a rate that is comfortable.

- Practice your competition fluid intake plan in training sessions.

- Get to know your sweat rate by weighing yourself before and after training sessions and competition.

- Water is an excellent fluid for low intensity and short duration sports.

- Sports drinks are ideally suited to high intensity 'stop-go' and endurance sports.

- Drink alcohol sensibly and assess the detrimental effects on your recovery.

Timing of Meal during Training

Melding a top-notch diet with stimulating exercise can be quite a challenge. Eating at different times, skipping meals, overeating, snacking in between, working out irregularly, suffering from injuries life gets in the way of our "healthy lifestyle plans." While flexibility can be a necessity and a virtue, keeping to a diet-and-exercise schedule has remarkable advantages. Eating regularly (5-7 times) throughout the day maintains proper blood sugar and energy levels, while regular exercise consistently burns consumed calories. Indeed, proper timing of nutrition and activity helps lay the foundation for optimizing physical results.

The benefits of coordinating workouts with food intake-both quality and quantity-your first question might focus on breakfast or some other fast-and-burn routine.

Some studies suggest intense physical activity such as running, swimming or bicycling on an empty stomach can increase fat burn and promote weight loss. However, many experts caution against pre-exercise fasting. Running on empty *may* help burn fat faster, but it won't leave enough energy for more rigorous training. It also can increase the risk of strains, sprains, stress fractures and other injuries from exercise-related fatigue. Furthermore, letting the body get too depleted may cause people to overeat afterward, undoing the benefits of exercising in the first place.

Therefore, adequate fueling before exercise is the better route to improving performance. This keeps the body fueled, providing steady energy and a satisfied stomach. Knowing the why, what and when to eat beforehand can make a significant difference in your training.

Training and Nutrient Timing before Events

A diet plan is crucial for maximizing daily workouts and recovery, especially in the lead-up to the big day. And no meal is more important than the one just before a race, big game or other athletic event. Choosing the wrong foods-eating or drinking too much, consuming too little or not timing a meal efficiently-can dramatically affect outcomes. Eating the ideal pre-race/event meal can help ensure that all of the hard training and dedication pay off. Similarly, maintaining an appropriate daily sports-nutrition plan creates the perfect opportunity for better results.

The main goal of a pre-event/workout meal is to replenish glycogen, the short-term storage form of carbohydrate. This supplies immediate energy needs and is crucial for morning workouts, as the liver is glycogen depleted from fueling the nervous system during sleep. The muscles, on the other hand, should be glycogen-loaded from proper recovery nutrition the previous day.

The body does not need a lot, but it needs something to prime the metabolism, provide a direct energy source, and allow for the planned intensity and duration of the given workout. But what is that something? That choice can make or break a workout. It is a good idea to experiment with several pre-exercise snacks/meals and stick with the few that work best under given circumstances.

The majority of nutrients in a preworkout meal should come from carbohydrates, as these macronutrients immediately fuel the body. Some protein should be consumed as well, but not a significant amount, as protein takes longer to digest and does not serve an immediate need for the beginning of an activity. Fat and dietary fiber also should be marginal to minimize the potential for gastrointestinal upset during the activity.

Research has demonstrated that the type of carbohydrate consumed does not directly affect performance across the board. Regular foods are ideal (e.g., a bagel with peanut butter), but convenience foods (energy bars or replacement shakes) may be helpful because you can determine the calories and the desired mix of carbohydrates, protein and fats. Exercisers might also supplement with a piece of fruit, glass of low-fat chocolate milk or another preferred carbohydrate, depending on needs.

Pre-exercise fluids are critical to prevent dehydration. To allow time to excrete excess fluid, start at least 4 hours before an activity and aim for an intake of 5-7 milliliters of water per kilogram of body weight. Before that, the athlete should drink enough water and fluids so that urine color is pale yellow and dilute-indicators of adequate hydration.

Timing is a huge consideration for preworkout nutrition. Too early and the meal is gone by the time the exercise begins; too late and the stomach is uncomfortably sloshing food around during the activity. Although body size, age, gender, metabolic rate, gastric motility and type of training are all meal-timing factors to consider, the ideal time for most people to eat is about 2-4 hours before activity. This much lead time can allow people to safely eat up to about 1,000 nutritious calories that will be ready for fueling the activity. If lead times are much shorter (a pre-7 a.m. workout, for example), eating a smaller meal of less than 300-400 calories about an hour before the workout can suffice.

It is customarily recommended that exercisers consume about 1 gram of carbohydrate per kilogram of body weight 1 hour before working out, and 2 g of carbohydrate per kg of body weight if 2 hours before exercise, and so on.

For a 150-pound athlete, that would equate to about 68 g (or 4-5 servings) of carbohydrate, 1 hour before exercise. For reference, 1 serving of a carbohydrate food contains about 15 g of carbohydrate. There are about 15 g of carbohydrate in each of the following: 1 slice of whole-grain bread, 1 orange, ½ cup cooked oatmeal, 1 small sweet potato or 1 cup low-fat milk. This 150-pound athlete could consider consuming: ½ cup oatmeal, 1 small apple, ½ cup low-fat yogurt and 4 ounces 100% fruit juice-all approximately 1 hour before working out.

It is generally best that anything consumed less than 1 hour before an event or workout be blended or liquid-such as a sports drink or smoothie-to promote rapid stomach emptying. Bear in mind that we are all individuals and our bodies will perform differently. It may take some study to understand what works best for you. Athletes should experiment with the size, timing and composition of pre-event/activity meals to determine what will be best tolerated.

Preworkout foods should not only be easily digestible, but also easily (and conveniently) consumed. A comprehensive preworkout nutrition plan should be evaluated based on the duration and intensity of exertion, the ability to supplement during the activity, personal energy needs, environmental conditions and the start time. For instance, a person who has a higher weight and is running in a longer-distance race likely needs a larger meal and supplemental nutrition during the event to maintain desired intensity.

Determining how much is too much or too little can be frustrating, but self-experimentation is crucial for success. The athlete ought to sample different prework-out meals during various training intensities as trials for what works. Those training for a specific event should simulate race day as closely as possible (time of day, conditions, etc.) when experimenting with several nutrition protocols to ensure optimal results.

Eating during Activity

Supplemental nutrition may not be necessary during shorter or less-intense activity bouts. Athletes may need to eat during the activity if exertion lasts more than roughly 1 hour and environmental conditions require glycogen to be restored to maintain intensity and duration. If so, carbohydrate consumption should begin shortly after the start of exercise. The general recommendation is based on the maximum rate of glucose absorption, which is to consume about 30-60 g of carbohydrate per hour during prolonged exercise. One popular sports-nutrition trend is to use multiple carb sources with different routes and rates of absorption to maximize the supply of energy to cells and lessen the risk of GI distress.

Sports drinks with 6-8% carbohydrate are quick and convenient sources of fluid, carbohydrate and electrolytes during extended bouts of exercise. Consuming 6-12 ounces of such drinks every 15-30 minutes during exercise has been shown to extend the exercise capacity of some athletes. However, athletes should refine these approaches according to their individual sweat rates, tolerances and exertion levels.

Some athletes prefer gels or chews to replace carbohydrates during extended activities. These sports supplements are formulated with a specific composition of nutrients to rapidly supply carbohydrates and electrolytes. Most provide about 25 g of carbohydrate per serving and should be consumed with water to speed digestion and prevent cramping.

Basics on Recovery

To improve fitness and endurance, we must anticipate the next episode of activity as soon as one exercise session ends. That means focusing on recovery, one of the most important-and often overlooked-aspects of proper sports nutrition.

An effective nutrition recovery plan supplies the right nutrients at the right time. Recovery is the body's process of adapting to the previous workload and strengthening itself for the next physical challenge. Nutritional components of recovery include carbohydrates to replenish depleted fuel stores, protein to help repair damaged muscle and develop new muscle tissue, and fluids and electrolytes to rehydrate.

A full, rapid recovery supplies more energy and hydration for the next workout or event, which improves performance and reduces the chance of injury. Rapid recovery is especially crucial during periods of heavy training and anytime two or more training sessions happen within 12 hours.

Training generally depletes muscle glycogen. The first 30 minutes or so after exercise provide an important opportunity for nutritional recovery due to factors like increased blood flow and insulin sensitivity, which boosts cellular glucose uptake and glycogen restoration.

To maximize muscle glycogen replacement, athletes should consume a carbohydrate-rich snack within this 30-minute window. The recommendation for rapidly replenishing glycogen stores is to take in foods providing 1.0-1.5 g of carbohydrate per kg of body weight within 30 minutes of extended exercise. For a 150-pound athlete, that equates to between 68 and 102 g of carbs (or ~ 4.5-6.5 servings of carbs) immediately after exercise. Since this can be difficult to consume in whole foods shortly after activity, liquid and bar supplements may be useful and convenient after exercise.

Ideally, athletes should repeat this carbohydrate load for 2-hour intervals for up to 6 hours, or transition to carbohydrate snacks and meals if another intense training session will occur within 24 hours. Consuming smaller amounts of carbohydrates more frequently may be prudent if the previous recommendation leaves the athlete feeling too full.

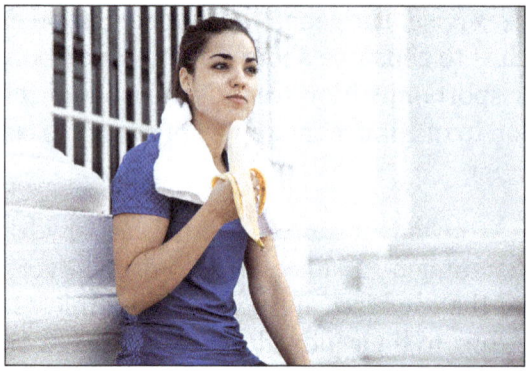 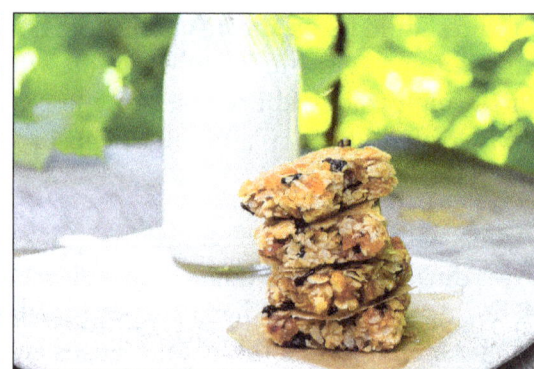

Eating Protein

Muscle tissue repair and muscle building are important for recovery. Whether you're focusing on endurance or strength training, taking in protein after a workout provides the amino acid building blocks needed to repair muscle fibers that get damaged and catabolized during exercise, and to promote the development of new muscle tissue. Although daily protein requirements vary among individuals, consuming 15-25 g of protein within 1 hour after exercise can maximize the muscle rebuilding and repair process.

Recent research has further demonstrated that a similar amount of protein (approximately 15-30 g) after resistance exercise may even benefit athletes on calorie-restricted diets who also want to maintain lean body mass. It is important to note that some literature emphasizing extremely high levels of protein intake-well beyond these recommendations-for strength training may be dated and lack quality research.

Rehydration

Virtually all weight lost during exercise is fluid, so weighing yourself (without clothes) before and after exercise can help gauge net fluid losses. Replace fluids by gradually (within 4-6 hours) drinking 16-24 fluid ounces of a recovery beverage, sports drink or water for every pound of weight lost. It is important to restore hydration status before the next exercise period. Rehydration will be more effective when sodium is included with the fluid and food consumed during recovery-especially in hot/humid conditions. However, water may be all you need if exercising for less than 1 hour at a low intensity.

Body's Timing Signals

While these recommendations are a good starting point, there are no absolute sports nutrition rules that satisfy everyone's needs so paying attention to how you feel during exercise and how diet affects performance is of utmost importance.

You may have to use different timing and alternate routines to create a nutrition and exercise combo that works best. Timing certainly is critical in sports nutrition, and optimizing that can make all the difference.

References

- During-exercise, nutrition: topendsports.com, Retrieved 25 February, 2019

- Recovery-nutrition, fuelling-recovery, factsheets: sportsdietitians.com.au, Retrieved 16 January, 2019

- Fluids-in-sport: sportsdietitians.com.au, Retrieved 29 March, 2019

- Nutrition-exercise-timing-is-everything, american-fitness-magazine-spring, issues, american-fitness-magazine: nasm.org, Retrieved 30 April, 2019

3

Sports Drinks, Foods and Supplements

Sports drinks are used to prevent dehydration and maintain the body's balance of fluids at an optimum level. Sports food, protein bars, energy gels, whey protein, soy protein, etc. are used by athletes for increasing the efficiency in their performance. This chapter discusses these sports drinks, foods and supplements in detail.

Sports Drinks

Sports drinks are beverages that are specially formulated to help people rehydrate during or after exercise. They are usually rich in carbohydrates - the most efficient source of energy.

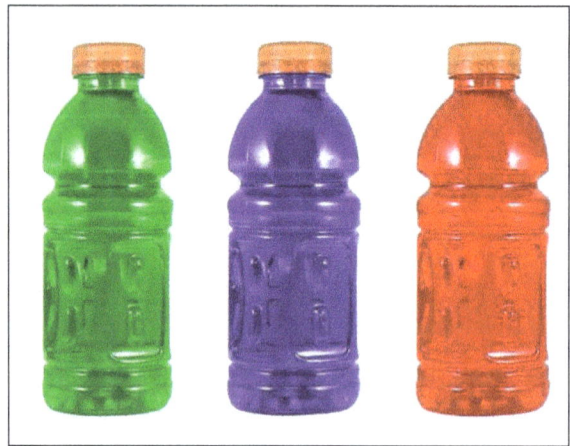

Sports drinks are often rich in carbohydrates.

As well as carbs, which are important in maintaining exercise and sport performance, sports drinks usually contain sweeteners and preservatives.

Sports drinks also contain electrolytes (minerals such as chloride, calcium, magnesium, sodium and potassium), which, along with body fluid, diminish as you exercise and sweat.

Replacing the electrolytes lost during training promotes proper rehydration, which is important in delaying the onset of fatigue during exercise.

Keeping rehyrdated is particularly important for people with diabetes who have an increased risk of dehydration due to high levels of blood glucose.

Types of Sport Drinks

There are three main types of sports drinks available.

Isotonic

Isotonic drinks contains similar concentrations of salt and sugar as in the human body:

- Quickly replaces fluids lost through sweating and supplies a boost of carbohydrate.

- The preferred choice for most athletes, including middle and long-distance running or those involved in team sports.

Hypertonic

Hypertonic drinks contain a higher concentration of salt and sugar than the human body.

- Normally consumed post-workout to supplement daily carbohydrate intake and top-up muscle glycogen stores.

- Can be taken during ultra distance events to meet the high energy demands, but must be used in conjunction with Isotonic drinks to replace lost fluids.

Hypotonic

Hypotonic drinks contain a lower concentration of salt and sugar than the human body.

- Quickly replaces fluids lost by sweating.

- Suitable for athletes who require fluid without a carbohydrate boost, e.g. gymnasts.

Most sports drinks are moderately isotonic, containing between 4 and 5 heaped teaspoons of sugar per five ounce (13 and 19 grams per 250 ml) serving.

Risk of Water Intoxication

While water is the best option for rehydrating your body, drinking excessive amounts can cause an imbalance of electrolytes in the body. This condition is known as water intoxication and although it is very rare, it can be fatal.

It occurs when large quantities of plain water are consumed to replace the fluid and electrolytes lost through heavy sweating caused by either hot weather or exercise, or a combination of the two.

For optimal performance, athletes should be hydrated and adequately fuelled during exercise. Although there are a wide range of beverages marketed with reference to sport or performance; sports drinks are specifically designed to provide the right balance of carbohydrate, electrolytes and fluid to adequately fuel exercise and provide fluid for hydration. When used appropriately they can result in performance benefits.

If drinking sports drink products in powdered form it is important to follow the manufacturer's instructions to ensure that the carbohydrate and electrolyte balance is optimal for gut absorption, fluid balance and fuel delivery. Incorrect preparation may lead to gastrointestinal discomfort and a negative impact on performance.

Table: The nutritional compotion of commercially available sprots drinks per 100 mL.

	Gatorade	Gatorade Endurance	Powerade	Powerade Zero	Maximus	Staminade
Energy	103 kJ	108 kJ	129 kJ	6.8 kJ	130 kJ	106 kJ
Protein	0g	0g	0g	0.05g	<1g	0 g
Fat – total	0g	0g	0g	0g	<1g	0 g
Saturated	0g	0g	0g	0.1g	<1g	0 g
Carbohydrate	6.0 g	6.2g	7.3g	0.1g	7.4g	6.0 g
– sucrose	5.5 g	5.7g	5.7g	0g	6.0g	4.4g
– glucose	0.5 g	0.5g	1.6g	n/a	1.6g	1.6g
Sodium	51 mg	84mg	28mg	51 mg	30 mg	37.9 mg
Potassium	22.5 mg	39.2mg	14.1 mg	n/a	30 mg	18.6 mg
Magnesium	n/a	1.4mg	n/a	n/a	4 mg	2.9 mg
Calcium	n/a	2.7mg	n/a	n/a	2 mg	–

Table: The nutritional compotion of commercially available sprots drinks per 1 L.

	Gatorade	Gatorade Endurance	Powerade	Powerade Zero	Maximus	Staminade
Energy	1030 kJ	1080 kJ	1290 kJ	68 kJ	1300 kJ	1060 kJ
Protein	0 g	0g	0g	0.5 g	<1g	0g
Fat – total	0 g	0g	0g	0g	<1 g	0g
Saturated	0 g	0g	0g	1g	<1 g	0g
Carbohydrate	60 g	62 g	73g	1g	74 g	60 g
– sucrose	55 g	57 g	57g	0g	60 g	44 g
– glucose	5 g	5 g	6g	n/a	16 g	16 g
Sodium	23 mg	84 0mg	28 0mg	510 mg	300 mg	379 mg
Potassium	225 mg	392 mg	141 mg	n/a	300 mg	186 mg
Magnesium	n/a	14 mg	n/a	n/a	40 mg	29 mg
Calcium	n/a	27 mg	n/a	n/a	20 mg	–

Ingredients of a Sports Drink

Carbohydrate

Carbohydrate can have performance benefits in a range of sporting events by providing a fuel source for muscles and the brain. Carbohydrate also contributes to the palatability (taste) of sports drinks. Most sports drinks contain 6-8% carbohydrate (6-8 g/L). Carbohydrate concentrations above this can impair gastric emptying and lead to gut upset during exercise and impair performance.

Electrolytes

Sports drinks include the electrolytes sodium and potassium. The sodium content of sports drinks encourages fluid intake by driving the thirst mechanism, while also increasing absorption and fluid retention. Sports drinks may also help with salt replacement for athletes who are heavy or salty sweaters. Low sodium drinks may not be suitable when speedy rehydration is necessary (i.e. when there is a need replace a fluid deficit in a short period of time). The addition of potassium to sports drinks helps maintain electrolyte balance and can assist with muscle contraction during exercise.

Flavour

Flavour is an important feature of sports drinks that helps to increase voluntary fluid intake (compared to water) during or after exercise.

Other Ingredients

Some beverages marketed as sports drinks have other added ingredients like vitamins, minerals, protein and herbal ingredients. These extra ingredients are likely to offer very little (if any) additional benefit over standard sports drink and may affect the palatability, and subsequently consumption of the fluid. Some sports drinks also contain caffeine which can have performance benefits.

Practical Applications

- Before exercise:

  Sports drinks may be useful before an event to fine tune fluid and fuel (carbohydrate) intake. The carbohydrate in sports drinks can increase carbohydrate availability, while the added sodium may reduce urine losses before exercise begins.

- During exercise:

  Sports drinks are primarily designed for use during exercise lasting more than 90 minutes by providing optimal fluid and fuel delivery. Sports drinks may allow athletes to perform for longer and more effectively in training and competition by providing energy to working muscles and the brain.

- Recovery:

  Sports drinks can help meet nutrition recovery goals by replacing fluids and electrolytes lost in sweat and helping to replenish glycogen stores. If there is limited time between training sessions or competition, drinks with higher sodium content may promote more effective rehydration. To meet all recovery goals, the ingestion of sports drinks should be complimented with foods and fluids that provide adequate carbohydrate, protein, and other nutrients essential for recovery.

Potential Side Effects

Gastrointestinal Upset

Excessive consumption of sports drink can cause gastrointestinal upset. It is recommended that athletes drink small amounts frequently (rather than a lot at once) and trial options during training.

Dental Health

Acidic foods and fluids are one of the factors linked to tooth enamel erosion. Sports drinks, together with fruit juice, soft drink, wine, beer, tea and coffee are all examples of acidic fluids. The use of sports drinks alone is unlikely to cause dental erosion. However, athletes who use large quantities of sports drinks for prolonged periods should pay extra attention to dental hygiene.

Diet Drinks

Diet sports drinks replenish electrolytes at a fraction of the calories of traditional sports drinks. Several commercially sold diet sports drinks are calorie free and include most of the electrolytes lost in sweat. Check the ingredient list for "electrolyte sources" to see which electrolytes are in the beverage. Sports drink brands also offer a low-calorie option with 30 calories and 7 grams of carbohydrates per 12-ounce serving, compared to the traditional sports drinks that contain 80 calories and 21 grams of carbohydrates.

Electrolyte Tablets and Powders

While diet sports drinks are convenient because they are ready to drink instantly, electrolyte tablets and powders are also convenient because they're portable. Leading electrolyte tablet brands transform a 16-ounce serving of water into an 8-calorie beverage with a balanced mix of electrolytes. Electrolyte powders are typically around 10 calories per packet, and some brands include immune-boosting vitamin C, zinc and selenium.

Coconut Water

Coconut water gives you a natural way to replenish electrolytes and carbohydrates for energy. This water inside young, green coconuts contains 45 to 50 calories and 9 to 11 grams of carbohydrates per 8-ounce serving. The nutrition facts are similar to low-calorie sports drinks, but the benefit of coconut water is the lack of preservatives.

Low-calorie Smoothies

Homemade smoothies are an affordable way to replenish electrolytes without preservatives and added sugar. A post-workout smoothie only requires a few ingredients: a fluid base, fruits and vegetables.

Water keeps smoothies low in calories. Add 1 dash of table salt to replenish about 155 mg of sodium. Two other fluid base options that don't require added salt are milk - cow's milk, soy milk or almond milk - or unsweetened coconut water.

Add fruit based on your preference; bananas, strawberries, blueberries and oranges supply high amounts of potassium. Leafy vegetables like spinach and kale supply electrolytes, vitamin A, C and K. Optional ingredients for extra protein include protein powder, peanut butter or almond butter.

Energy Drink

An energy drink is a type of drink containing sugar and stimulant compounds, usually caffeine, which is marketed as providing mental and physical stimulation (marketed as "energy", but distinct from food energy). They may or may not be carbonated and may also contain other sweeteners, herbal extracts, taurine, and amino acids. They are a subset of the larger group of energy products, which includes bars and gels, and distinct from sports drinks, which are advertised to enhance sports performance. There are many brands and varieties in this drink category.

Coffee, tea and other naturally caffeinated drinks are usually not considered energy drinks. Other soft drinks such as cola may contain caffeine, but are not considered energy drinks either. Some alcoholic drinks, such as Buckfast Tonic Wine, contain caffeine and other stimulants. According to the Mayo Clinic, it is safe for the typical healthy adult to consume a total of 400 mg of caffeine a day. This has been confirmed by a panel of the European Food Safety Authority, which also concludes that a caffeine intake of up to 400 mg per day does not raise safety concerns for adults. According to the ESFA this is equivalent to 4 cups of coffee (90 mg each) or 2 1/2 standard cans (250 ml) of energy drink (160 mg each/80 mg per serving).

Energy drinks have the effects caffeine and sugar provide, but there is little or no evidence that the wide variety of other ingredients have any effect. Most effects of energy drinks on cognitive performance, such as increased attention and reaction speed, are primarily due to the presence of caffeine. Other studies ascribe those performance improvements to the effects of the combined ingredients. Advertising for energy drinks usually features increased muscle strength and endurance, but there is still no scientific consensus to support these claims. Energy drinks have been associated with health risks, such as an increased rate of injury when usage is combined with alcohol, and excessive or repeated consumption can lead to cardiac and psychiatric conditions. Populations at-risk for complications from energy drink consumption include youth, caffeine-naïve or caffeine-sensitive, pregnant, competitive athletes and people with underlying cardiovascular disease.

Uses

Energy drinks are marketed to provide the benefits among health effects of caffeine along with benefits from the other ingredients they contain. Health experts agree that energy drinks which contain caffeine do improve alertness. The consumption of alcoholic drinks combined with energy drinks is a common occurrence on many college campuses. The alcohol industry has recently been criticized for marketing cohesiveness of alcohol and energy drinks. The combination of the two in college students is correlated to students experiencing alcohol-related consequences, and several health risks.

There is no reliable evidence that other ingredients in energy drinks provide further benefits, even though the drinks are frequently advertised in a way that suggests they have unique benefits. The dietary supplements in energy drinks may be purported to provide produce benefits, such as for vitamin B12, but no claims of using supplements to enhance health in otherwise normal people have been verified scientifically. Various marketing organizations such as Red Bull and Monster have described energy drinks by saying their product "gives you wings", is "scientifically formulated", or is a "killer energy brew". Marketing of energy drinks has been particularly directed towards teenagers, with manufacturers sponsoring or advertising at extreme sports events and music concerts, and targeting a youthful audience through social media channels.

When mixed with alcohol, either as a prepackaged caffeinated alcoholic drink, a mixed drink, or just a drink consumed alongside alcohol, energy drinks are often consumed in social settings.

Effects

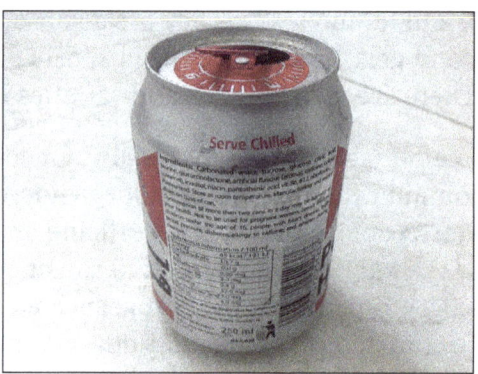

A health warning on a can of the energy drink.

Energy drinks have the effects caffeine and sugar provide, but there is little or no evidence that the wide variety of other ingredients have any effect. Most of the effects of energy drinks on cognitive performance, such as increased attention and reaction speed, are primarily due to the presence of caffeine. Advertising for energy drinks usually features increased muscle strength and endurance, but there is little evidence to support this in the scientific literature.

A caffeine intake of 400 mg per day is considered as safe from the European Food Safety Authority (EFSA). Adverse effects associated with caffeine consumption in amounts greater than 400 mg include nervousness, irritability, sleeplessness, increased urination, abnormal heart rhythms (arrhythmia), and dyspepsia. Consumption also has been known to cause pupil dilation. Caffeine dosage is not required to be on the product label for food in the United States, unlike drugs, but most (although not all) place the caffeine content of their drinks on the label anyway, and some advocates are urging the FDA to change this practice.

Energy drinks could be causing some major damage to the community consuming them: Youth. As the youth continues to consume more and more sugar they are being provided with more health issues such as Type 2 Diabetes, Cavities, Early onset Rheumatoid Arthritis, Heart disease, heart attacks, and strokes, and more. Typically these are issues that come around later in life, which are now affecting the youth of today's society.

With Alcohol

Combined use of caffeine and alcohol may increase the rate of alcohol-related injury. Energy drinks can mask the influence of alcohol, and a person may misinterpret their actual level of intoxication.

Since caffeine and alcohol are both diuretics, combined use increases the risk of dehydration, and the mixture of a stimulant (caffeine) and depressant (alcohol) sends contradictory messages to the nervous system and can lead to increased heart rate and palpitations. Although people decide to drink energy drinks with alcohol with the intent of counteracting alcohol intoxication, many others do so to hide the taste of alcohol. However, in the 2015, the EFSA concluded, that "Consumption of other constituents of energy drinks at concentrations commonly present in such beverages would not affect the safety of single doses of caffeine up to 200 mg." Also the consumption of alcohol, leading to a blood alcohol content of about 0.08%, would, according to the EFSA, not affect the safety of single doses of caffeine up to 200 mg. Up to these levels of intake, caffeine is unlikely to mask the subjective perception of alcohol intoxication.

Health Problems

Excessive consumption of energy drinks can have serious health effects resulting from high caffeine and sugar intakes, particularly in children, teens, and young adults. Excessive energy drink consumption may disrupt teens' sleep patterns and may be associated with increased risk-taking behavior. Excessive or repeated consumption of energy drinks can lead to cardiac problems, such as arrhythmias and heart attacks, and psychiatric conditions such as anxiety and phobias. In Europe, energy drinks containing taurine and caffeine have been associated with the deaths of athletes. Reviews have noted that caffeine content was not the only factor, and that the cocktail of other ingredients in energy drinks made them more dangerous than drinks whose only stimulant was caffeine.

Research suggests that emergency department (ED) visits are on the increase. In 2005, there were 1,494 emergency department visits related to energy drink consumption in the United States; whereas, in 2011, energy drinks were linked to 20,783 emergency department visits. During this period of increase, male consumers consistently had a higher likelihood of visiting the emergency department over their female counterparts. Research trends also show that emergency department visits are caused mainly by adverse reactions to the drinks. In 2011, there were 14,042 energy drink-related hospital visits. Misuse and abuse of these caffeinated drinks also cause a significant amount of emergency department visits. By 2011, there were 6,090 visits to the ED due to misuse/abuse of the drinks. In many cases 42% of patients had mixed energy drinks with another stimulant, and in the other 58% of cases the energy drink was the only thing that had been consumed. Several studies suggest that energy drinks may be a gateway drug.

Variants

Energy Shots

Energy shots are a specialized kind of energy drink. Whereas most energy drinks are sold in cans or bottles, energy shots are usually sold in smaller 50 ml bottles. Energy shots can contain the same total amount of caffeine, vitamins or other functional ingredients as their larger versions, and may be considered concentrated forms of energy drinks. The marketing of energy shots generally focuses on their convenience and availability as a low-calorie "instant" energy drink that can be taken in one swallow (or "shot"), as opposed to energy drinks that encourage users to drink an entire can, which may contain 250 calories or more. A common energy shot is 5-hour Energy which contains B vitamins and caffeine in an amount similar to a cup of coffee.

Caffeinated Alcoholic Drink

Energy drinks such as Red Bull are often used as mixers with alcoholic drinks, producing mixed drinks such as Vodka Red Bull which are similar to but stronger than rum and coke with respect to the amount of caffeine that they contain. Sometimes this is configured as a bomb shot, such as the Jägerbomb or the *F-Bomb* — Fireball Cinnamon Whisky and Red Bull.

Caffeinated alcoholic drinks are also sold in some countries in a wide variety of formulations.

Chemistry

Supplement Facts		
Serving Size 8.0 fl.oz. (240 mL)		
Servings Per Container: 2		
Amount Per Serving		**% Daily Value**
Calories	**100**	
Total Carb	**27g**	**9%***
Sugars	27g	†
Riboflavin Vit B2	1.7mg	100%
Niacin Vit B3	20mg	100%
Vitamin B6	2mg	100%
Vitamin B12	.6mcg	100%
Sodium	180mg	8%
Taurine	1000mg	†
Panax Ginseng	200mg	†
Energy Blend	2500mg	†
L-Carnitine, Glucose, Caffeine, Guarana, Inositol, Glucuronolactone, Maltodextrin		
*Percent Daily Values are based on a 2000 calorie diet. † Daily Value not established.		

A Nutrition facts label for an energy drink.

Energy drinks generally contain methylxanthines (including caffeine), B vitamins, carbonated water, and high-fructose corn syrup (for non-diet versions). Other common ingredients are guarana, yerba mate, açaí, and taurine, plus various forms of ginseng, maltodextrin, inositol, carnitine, creatine, glucuronolactone, sucralose or ginkgo biloba. The sugar in non-diet energy drinks is food energy, while there is no scientific evidence that addition of other ingredients has any effect on human health.

In the United States, the caffeine content of energy drinks is in the range of 40 to 250 mg per 8 fluid ounce (237 ml) serving. The Food and Drug Administration recommends that 400 mg per day is safe for adults, while 1200 mg per day can be toxic.

Recovery Drinks

While the list of health benefits exercise provides is lengthy, exercise also depletes your body of important nutrients and energy. Consuming a recovery drink that contains the right types of nutrients at the right times following your workouts can make a considerable difference in your exercise results and overall health.

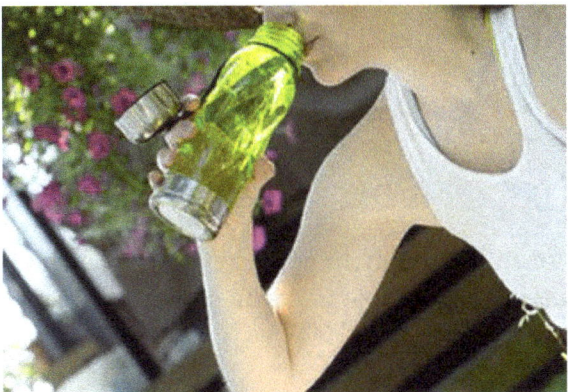

Woman during her morning workout.

Timing

Recovery drinks help replenish fluids and energy lost during your workout and prepare you for your next workout. For the first two hours after exercise your liver produces glycogen, the short-term storage form of glucose, at one-and-a-half times the normal rate. This is the best time to have a high-carbohydrate recovery drink. Consuming carbohydrates immediately after exercise also stimulates your pancreas to release insulin, which tells your cells to absorb glucose. During the next four hours glycogen production remains elevated, but gradually slows.

Fatigue

If you exercise twice a day, consuming a carbohydrate-based recovery drink will ensure sufficient energy to fuel you through your second workout. It will also help you avoid potential injury and progress more rapidly toward your exercise goals. With time and regular training, your glycogen storage capacity increases by up to 20 percent. This translates to greater endurance and better performance in your chosen sport. Aim for 1.5 grams of carbohydrate for every kilogram of your body weight in the first 30 minutes after exercise and every two hours for the first four hours to six hours.

Aerobic Capacity

Your recovery drink can satisfy both your glucose requirements and your chocolate cravings. According to the University of Texas at Austin Department of Kinesiology and Health Education, low-fat chocolate milk is an ideal post-workout recovery drink for promoting more lean muscle mass and less fat. Protein in chocolate milk makes it a superior recovery drink to those with carbohydrates alone. It can also increase your strength, speed and aerobic capacity - a measure of your body's ability to use oxygen - by as much as two times.

Body Composition

A study published found that a recovery drink containing carbohydrate, protein and ribose - one of the building blocks of ATP, an important energy-carrying molecule - may improve body composition in endurance athletes. Participants, all males in their mid 20s, consumed the test drink immediately after exercising five days per week for eight weeks. Results showed reduced body fat percentage within the first three to six weeks. Body weight, aerobic capacity and endurance did not change significantly in response to the recovery drink in this study.

Sports Foods

Sports foods are specially formulated to help people achieve specific nutritional or sporting performance goals. They are intended to supplement the diet of sports people rather than be the only or main source of nutrition.

To meet the specific dietary requirements of sports people, this Standard allows the addition of substances that are not permitted or are restricted in other foods as well as higher levels of some vitamins and minerals. This means that these foods are not suitable for children or pregnant women.

The labels of sports foods must:

- Say 'formulated supplementary sports food'.

- Indicate that they are not a sole source of nutrition and should be consumed in conjunction with a nutritious diet and an appropriate physical training or exercise program.

- Provide directions stating the recommended quantity and frequency of intake of the food and state the recommended consumption of the food in one day.

- State that that they are 'Not suitable for children under 15 years of age or pregnant women: Should only be used under medical or dietetic supervision'.

The labels of sports foods must also provide the same information required on nearly all packaged foods. For example, a nutrition information panel and a list of the ingredients must be provided on the labels of most sports foods.

Other foods used by sports people are not regulated specifically as sports foods, such as general purpose foods (e.g. pasta, bananas, meat) and electrolyte drinks.

Food for Energy

Starchy and other forms of carbohydrate provide a source of energy for your body to perform at its best, no matter what your sport or activity.

In general, the more you exercise, the more carbohydrate you need to include in your daily meals and around exercise.

A demanding exercise regime will use up your stored energy from carbohydrate quickly, so include some carbohydrate in most of your meals.

A diet low in carbohydrate can lead to a lack of energy during exercise, loss of concentration, and delayed recovery.

If you wish to adopt a lower carbohydrate diet for your sport, you should seek specialist advice.

Healthy sources of carbohydrate include:

- Wholegrain bread.
- Wholegrain breakfast cereals (including some cereal bars).
- Brown rice.
- Wholewheat pasta.
- Potatoes (with skins on).
- Fruit, including dried and tinned fruit.

Food for Muscles

Eating protein-rich foods alone won't build big muscles.

Muscle is gained through a combination of muscle-strengthening exercise, and a diet that contains protein and sufficient energy from a balance of carbohydrates and fats.

Not all the protein you eat is used to build new muscle. If you overeat protein, the excess will be used mostly for energy once your body has what it needs for muscle repair.

Most fitness enthusiasts can get enough protein from a healthy, varied diet without having to increase their protein intake significantly.

Healthy sources of protein:

- Beans, peas and lentils.
- Cheese, yoghurt and milk.
- Fish, including oily fish like salmon or mackerel.
- Eggs.
- Tofu, tempeh and other plant-based meat-alternatives.
- Lean cuts of meat and mince.
- Chicken and other poultry.

A source of protein should be included at most mealtimes to optimise muscle building.

Taking in protein before and after a workout has been shown to help kickstart the muscle repair process.

Training protein snacks:

- Milk of all types – but lower-fat types contain less energy.
- Unsweetened soy drink.

- Natural dairy yoghurt of all types – including Greek yoghurt and kefir.

- Soy yoghurt and other plant-based alternatives.

- Unsalted mixed nuts and seeds.

- Unsweetened dried fruit.

- Boiled eggs.

- Hummus with carrot and celery sticks.

Food before Sport and Exercise

You should allow about three hours before you exercise after having a main meal, such as breakfast or lunch.

An hour before exercising, having a light snack that contains some protein, and is higher in carbohydrate and lower in fat, is a good choice to help you perform during your training and recover afterwards.

Choose a snack that you'll digest quickly, like:

- Porridge.

- Fruit, such as a banana.

- A slice of wholegrain bread spread thinly with a nut butter.

- A plain or fruit scone with low-fat cheese.

- Yoghurt or non-dairy alternatives.

- Cottage cheese and crackers.

- A glass of milk or non-dairy alternatives.

Snacks to Avoid before Exercise

These types of food may cause stomach discomfort if eaten just before exercising.

Fatty foods, like:

- Chips or french fries.

- Avocados.

- Olives.

- Crisps.

- Full-fat cheeses.

- Large amounts of nuts.

High-fibre foods, like:

- Raw vegetables.

- High-fibre cereals.

- Raw nuts and seeds.

Food is the fuel that helps athletes perform their best. Without it, endurance, strength and overall performance will be down. If you want to get the most out of your workouts and athletic capabilities, your diet should be a top priority in your fitness efforts.

As your body puts out energy through exercise and training, you need to replenish those lost nutrients, which can be done by choosing the right foods.

Berries

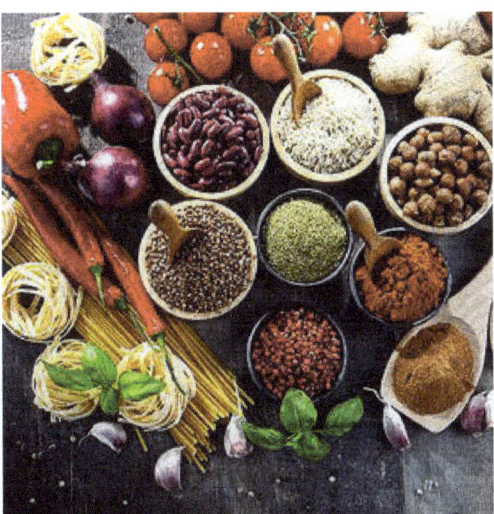

Blackberries, raspberries and blueberries are just a handful of the delicious berries that are rich in antioxidants, which need to be replenished after physical activity. Darker berries contain phytochemicals and other protective elements that prevent oxidative stress that occurs in the body during strenuous activities. They also preserve muscle strength as you age, so they're good for the long term.

Salmon

This oily fish is packed with lean, muscle-building protein and omega-3 fatty acids, which reduces the inflammation that can happen with continual athletic activity. It is also a natural artery cleanser, helping to prevent heart disease, which can affect even the most active people.

Beans/Legumes

Vegetarians and meat eaters alike can get their fill of plant-based protein by eating beans and legumes. Black beans, pinto beans, kidney beans, lima beans. Unlike meat, beans and legumes don't have saturated fat and contain fiber, which will help you feel fuller longer.

Bananas

Bananas are a low-calorie, excellent source of natural electrolytes, which need to be replaced after a workout or sporting event. They're also high in potassium, which makes them the perfect post-event snack. Eating one banana will help you regulate your fluid intake. It will also protect you from muscle spasms or cramps.

Cruciferous Vegetables

Dark, leafy greens such as spinach and kale, as well as broccoli, cauliflower and brussel sprouts are rich in antioxidants, vitamins and minerals to boost your athletic abilities. They also contain high levels of vitamins A, K and B6, and calcium and iron, all of which protect the body against inflammation. Iron also means more oxygen being supplied to working muscles. Kale contains carotenoids and flavonoids, two power antioxidants, and fiber, which helps lower cholesterol.

Nuts

Nuts are high in protein and healthy fats, making them a mainstay in athletes' diets. Eaten with carbs, they help level out your blood sugar and sustain the carbs over a longer period of time, rather than burning them off right away. They're also easier to digest and don't upset your stomach. Another plant-based protein, nuts are rich in fiber and antioxidants like vitamin E. The anti-inflammatory nutrients found in nuts makes them great for bone health, which is needed by every athlete. They also lower the bad cholesterol, which is good for heart health.

Milk

Milk is loaded with carbs and protein, which makes it a great post-workout drink for muscle recovery. The caffeine found in chocolate dilates the blood vessels, helping them to relax after a workout. Interestingly enough, when carbs and protein are consumed together, muscle tissues repair themselves more quickly than they do when consumed separately.

Sweet Potatoes

Sweet potatoes are rich in vitamins A and C, both antioxidants that remove free radicals from your body. They lower blood pressure, which is important for athletes to their heart health when participating in sports. They're high in vitamin and mineral content and contain the levels of potassium, iron, manganese and copper athletes need for healthy muscles.

Oatmeal

Oatmeal is an excellent source of energy carbs for athletes and is high in fiber, helping you feel fuller, longer. It's 100 percent whole grain, helping to lower your risk of heart disease. If you're looking to gain weight, oatmeal is a delicious way to help you achieve your goal weight.

Whey Protein

Whey protein contains the essential amino acids. Quickly absorbed by the body, it lacks fat and cholesterol, which makes it an ideal formula for athletes to consume. Whey contains the levels of protein and amino acids necessary to rebuild muscles and protects against muscle breakdown.

Flaxseed, Olive and Coconut Oil

The monounsaturated fats found in olive oil have anti-inflammatory properties, which athletes need when putting so much stress on their bodies. Flaxseed oil contains omega-3s, which is also anti-inflammatory, to help recover quickly with bumps and bruises. It also contains fiber and protein. Coconut oil is filled with medium chain triglycerides (MCTs), which can help with your endurance during a grueling workout. The MCTs in coconut oil can also help with metabolism and energy from fat.

Cherries

An antioxidant-filled fruit, cherries aid in preventing muscle pain after running. It reduces inflammation, which is what causes such striking pain. Many athletes consume cherry juice as another way to lower exercise-based muscle damage, which can help reduce soreness.

Sport Energy Bars

Athletes consume energy bars for a variety of reasons, including fuel during a workout or race; using a bar as a meal replacement; and noshing on a bar as a snack. Endurance workout and race durations can vary wildly from around 20 minutes to 17 hours or more.

The field of sports nutrition works to design products that allow us to continue to work out and perform at higher intensity for longer. Energy bars are primarily composed of carbohydrates, with smaller amounts of protein and fat, while energy gels and chews are usually just carbohydrates. These all are convenient forms of sugar that digest quickly to provide you with energy. They are designed to work with our energy systems and specifically support the aerobic system, which burns on carbohydrates.

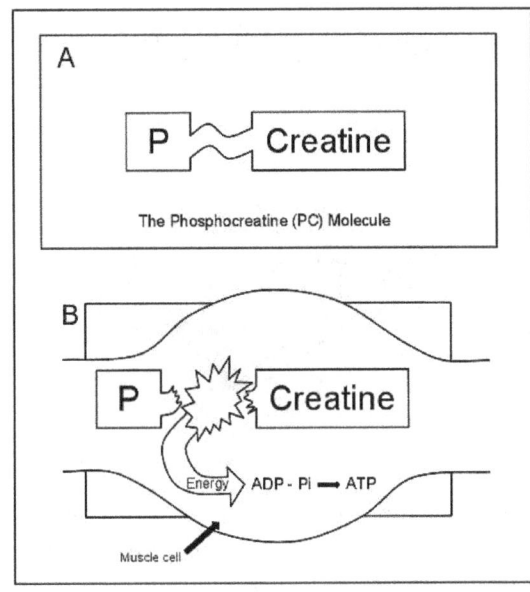

Energy Systems of the Body

We have three different systems in our bodies to create more ATP:

Creatine phosphate (CP) system, also sometimes known as the ATP-PC system. CP is stored in our cells and can be rapidly converted into ATP and burned., it takes a second to start burning but does not last a long time. On average someone sprinting will burn through their CP stores in fifteen to thirty seconds.

Anaerobic system, also sometimes called the glycolytic system. This involves burning carbohydrates without oxygen. It allows us relatively quick fuel, but at the expense of simultaneously creating lactic acid. It is an unsustainable energy system.

The aerobic system Carbohydrates are converted with oxygen to produce ATP. This is a very efficient system and can operate for a long time. But our bodies have limited storage for carbohydrates, which are stored as glycogen. The human body holds roughly 2,000 calories of glycogen. This is stored in three places - our blood stream (blood sugar), muscles, and liver. Roughly 400 grams can be stored in the muscles and 100 grams in the liver, with a minimal amount in the blood stream. As our muscles deplete their glycogen, the liver releases its stores that are then made available for muscles to burn.

Ideal Situations for Consuming Energy Bars

If you have ideal conditions and your storage levels are near 100% you have enough fuel for roughly twenty miles of running or several hours of moderate intensity exercise. Eating some version of an energy product will give you additional sugar to burn so you can continue to operate at the same intensity level and keep running. If you don't supplement with food, you will have to utilize primarily your ability to burn fat, but this process works at a slower rate and will force you to slow down.

Energy products can also be used for high intensity exercise or shorter duration training sessions.

Unsuitable Situations for Consuming Energy Bars

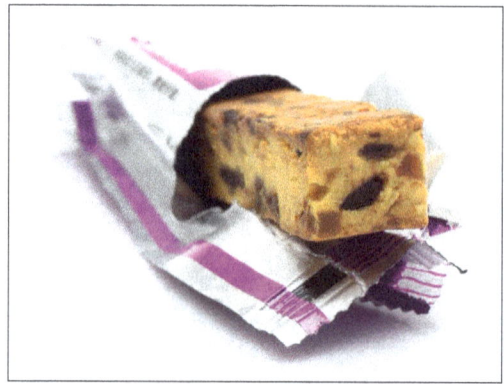

Energy bars should not be a snack during the day. You wouldn't put jet fuel in your car, so don't use jet fuel when you plan on sitting on your butt. Energy products are also not a substitute for regular food. They should be used as sports nutrition and for when you are going to be active.

Protein Bars

Protein bars are nutrition bars that contain a high proportion of protein to carbohydrates/fats.

Dietary Purpose

Protein bars are targeted to people who primarily want a convenient source of protein that doesn't require preparation (unless homemade). There are different kinds of food bars to fill different purposes. Energy bars provide the majority of their food energy (calories) in carbohydrate form. Meal replacement bars are intended to replace the variety of nutrients in a meal. Protein bars are usually lower in carbs than energy bars, lower in vitamins and dietary minerals than meal replacement bars, and significantly higher in protein than either. Protein bars are mainly used by athletes or exercise enthusiasts for muscle building.

Protein Bar Niche

In addition to other nutrients, the human body needs protein to build muscles. In the fitness and medical fields it is generally accepted that protein after exercise helps build the muscles used. Whey protein is one of the most popular protein sources used for athletic performance. Other protein sources include egg albumen protein and casein, which is typically known as the slow digestive component of milk protein. Vegan protein bars contain only plant proteins from sources like peas, brown rice, hemp, and soybeans.

Issues

Sugar Content

Protein bars may contain high levels of sugar and sometimes are called "candy bars in disguise." To keep calories and carbohydrate content relatively low, many protein bars contain sugar alcohol as sweetener.

Supplementation Controversy

There is a disagreement over the amount of protein required for active individuals and athletic performance. Some research shows that protein supplementation is not necessary. Athletes generally consume higher levels of protein as compared to the general population for muscular hypertrophy and to reduce lean body mass lost during weight loss.

The American Dietetic Association, Dietitians of Canada, and American College of Sports Medicine supports higher protein intake for athletes in order to enhance athletic performance and recovery.

Protein bars include isolated protein from one or more sources; for example, milk, soy or eggs. They can include other ingredients as well that offer carbohydrates, fats, vitamins or minerals to bolster your intake of these nutrients, and they typically come in a variety of flavors for improved taste. The quality of the protein, as well as the amount and quality of added ingredients, influences whether these supplements might help or hinder your nutrition and overall health.

Advantages

When protein bars include high-quality protein – such as from soy or animal sources – they contribute essential amino acids to your diet to help you build and maintain muscle mass, synthesize immune and red blood cells, repair wounds or damaged tissues and manufacture both hormones and enzymes. They can also supply energy in the form of carbohydrates or fats, as well as vitamins or minerals for supporting your overall health. Because they need no refrigeration or preparation, they make a convenient on-the-go snack or small meal replacement. Depending on your fitness goals, they can offer a boost of protein for relatively few calories when you are trying to lose weight, or additional nutrients to augment your regular meal plan when you are adding to your body mass.

Disadvantages

Even protein bars packed with ingredients cannot replace all the nutrients found in whole-food sources. Relying on protein bars for a significant proportion of your food intake can deny you the benefits of the vitamins, minerals, heart-healthy fats, phytochemicals and fiber abundant in natural foods. In addition, the convenience of protein bars comes at a price. Sports nutritionist Nancy Clark estimates protein bars can cost up to three times more than whole foods containing an equivalent amount of protein. If your regular food intake supplies sufficient protein and energy to meet your fitness needs, consuming protein bars can also add unwanted calories to your diet.

Energy Gels

Energy gels are carbohydrate gels that provide energy for exercise and promote recovery, commonly used in endurance events such as running, cycling, and triathlons. Energy gels are also referred to as endurance gels, sports gels, nutritional gels, and carbohydrate gels. They come in small, single-serve plastic packets. Each packet has a strip with a small notch at the top that can be peeled off to reveal an opening through which the gel can be consumed.

Sports energy gels emerged in the United Kingdom in 1986 as a "convenient, prewrapped, portable" way to deliver carbohydrates during endurance events. Gels have a gooey texture and are sometimes referred to as "goo" generically. The gel Leppin Squeezy was distributed at the Hawaii Ironman Triathlon in 1988. Once considered a "cult product in clear packaging", energy gel products are now marketed in fancy packaging and come in a variety of flavors. The energy gel market grew during the 1990s, as professional athletes began endorsing products. Manufacturers generally encourage the consumption of multiple packets, with water, when participating in endurance events.

Nutritional Behavior

Once consumed, the carbohydrates found in the gels are absorbed into the blood to supply the body with calories and nutrients to fuel exercise activity by helping to delay muscular fatigue, raise blood sugar levels, and enhance performance. Most energy gels have no fat, fiber, or protein, so they can be digested quickly. They contain mainly sugars and maltodextrins, which make them similar to sports drinks without the water. Since simple carbohydrates slow down gastric emptying and can cause gastrointestinal distress in athletes, there are attempts to create new categories of energy gels made with complex, long chain carbohydrates and fat. There are also gels with extras such as ginseng and other herbs, amino acids, vitamins, and Coenzyme Q10. Caffeine can be found in some gels as well.

Use

The recommended use of an energy gel is 15 minutes before starting and 30–45 minutes after starting the endurance exercise. The first gel prior to exercise may be skipped in favor of a high carbohydrate snack instead. Energy gels are then to be used every 30–45 minutes during exercise. The notch can be peeled off at the top and an intake of energy gel is recommended to be followed with a drink of water to avoid risk of dehydration. This is especially important for gels with high simple carbohydrate content. These gels create hyperosmolar gastric content which prevents carbohydrate absorption and gastrointestinal distress. For this reason, energy gels with low sugar content are frequently called "hydrogels". The exact intake of the gel varies for every athlete depending on their metabolism, body weight, and fitness level.

Advantages of Energy Gels

- There are added ingredients such as electrolytes, that help the athlete by bringing the body into balance while it is being stressed and dehydrated.

- Ginseng, amino acids, vitamins and Coenzyme Q10 are also added to some gels to aid performance. Gu's Roctane contains an Amino Acid Blend of Histidine, Leucine, Valine, and Isoleucine to reduce acid build-up and the Alpha-Ketoglutarate (OKG) reduces muscle damage.

- Caffeine can be added to some gels for energy.

- Convenient to open with the easy to peel notch.

- Gels can be carried conveniently in a pocket and they are not heavy.

- Gels are absorbed and digested easily and have an immediate effect.

Disadvantages of Energy Gels

- If the energy gel is not taken with water, it can lead to dehydration.

- Some gels do not taste nice.

- Gels may cause heartburn or reflux.

- If the gel is messed, it is sticky.

- Purchasing a few gels is more costly than sports drinks.

Energy gels are convenient for endurance athletes but they must find the gel flavour and type that works for them. There are many energy gels to choose from and athletes should experiment with various flavours. After an endurance race, athletes should rehydrate with water and eat a meal containing protein to facilitate muscle recovery.

Dietary Supplement

The term "dietary supplement" describes a broad and diverse category of products that you eat or drink to support good health and supplement the diet. Dietary supplements are not medicines, nor should they be considered a substitute for food.

Dietary ingredients can be one or a combination of any of the following:

- Vitamin.

- Mineral.

- Herb or other botanical.

- Amino acid (the individual building blocks of a protein).

- Concentrate, metabolite, constituent, or extract.

Although some herbal and mineral compounds have been used for hundreds of years to treat health conditions, today dietary supplement manufacturers are not legally allowed to say their products cure, treat or prevent disease. Supplement makers can say their products support health or contribute to well-being.

Except for new dietary ingredients, dietary supplement manufacturers do not need to prove that a product is safe or effective to be able to sell them. And, unlike medicines, which are required to meet USP standards to help ensure product consistency across multiple manufacturers, USP standards are voluntary for dietary supplements.

Dietary supplements are widely available in health food stores, drug stores, grocery stores, fitness centers and online and they come in many forms including: 2 piece capsules, soft gels, tablets, bottles of liquid, powders and gummies.

Dietary Supplements and Sports Performance

Sports success is dependent primarily on genetic endowment in athletes with morphologic, psychologic, physiologic and metabolic traits specific to performance characteristics vital to their sport. Such genetically-endowed athletes must also receive optimal training to increase physical power, enhance mental strength, and provide a mechanical advantage. However, athletes often attempt to go beyond training and use substances and techniques, often referred to as ergogenics, in attempts to gain a competitive advantage. Pharmacological agents, such as anabolic steroids and amphetamines, have been used in the past, but such practices by athletes have led to the establishment of anti-doping legislation and effective testing protocols to help deter their use. Thus, many athletes have turned to various dietary strategies, including the use of various dietary supplements (sports supplements), which they presume to be effective, safe and legal.

Dietary supplements are used by athletes worldwide. In the United States, the Dietary Supplement Health and Education Act has defined dietary supplements as something added to the diet, mainly (1) vitamins, (2) minerals, (3) amino acids, (4) herbs or botanicals, and (5) metabolites/constituents/extracts, or combination of any of these ingredients. In addition to actual food products targeted to athletes and physically-active individuals, numerous companies have marketed dietary supplements to athletes, often with the claim that sports performance may be enhanced.

Vitamins: Ergogenic Theory

Vitamins function in the human body as metabolic regulators, influencing a number of physiological processes important to exercise or sport performance. For example, many of the B-complex vitamins are involved in processing carbohydrate and fats for energy production, an important consideration during exercise of varying intensity. Several B vitamins are also essential to help form hemoglobin in red blood cells, a major determinant of oxygen delivery to the muscles during aerobic endurance exercise. Additionally, vitamins C and E function as antioxidants, important for preventing oxidative damage to cellular and subcellular structure and function during exercise training, theoretically optimizing preparation for competition.

Vitamin deficiencies can certainly impair exercise performance. A daily intake of less than one-third of the RDA for several of the B vitamins (B_1, B_2 and B_6) and vitamin C, even when other vitamins are supplemented in the diet, may lead to a significant decrease in VO_2max and the anaerobic threshold in less than four weeks. However, most studies report that athletes who consume high-calorie diets that contain the RDA of all nutrients have few vitamin or mineral deficiencies. Nevertheless, recent survey data indicate that vitamins are the most commonly used dietary supplements among various athletic groups. Can vitamin supplementation above that provided by an adequate, healthy, balanced diet enhance sport or exercise performance?

Studies have been conducted to evaluate the ergogenic potential of virtually every individual vitamin, as well as clusters of vitamins and related substances, including the B-complex vitamins, Multivitamin or mineral compounds, and antioxidants.

B Vitamins and Choline

As many of the B vitamins are involved in the metabolism of carbohydrate, fat and protein, their ergogenic potential has been studied individually and in combination. In general, although a deficiency of the B vitamins may impair both aerobic and anaerobic exercise performance, supplementation has not been shown to enhance performance in well-nourished individuals. Niacin supplementation may influence fat metabolism, blocking the release of free fatty acids (FFA) from adipose tissue and increasing reliance on carbohydrate utilization, possibly leading to premature depletion of muscle glycogen. Some research has indicated that excess niacin supplementation may actually impair aerobic endurance performance. Vitamins B_1, B_6 and B_{12} are believed to affect the formation of serotonin, an important neurotransmitter involved in relaxation. Some research with large doses (60–200 times the RDA) of these vitamins has shown increases in fine motor control and performance in pistol shooting. Others have suggested that the beneficial effect was related to the role of these vitamins in promoting the development of neurotransmitters that induce relaxation. Additional research is merited to evaluate these effects on performance in precision sports dependent on fine motor control. However, it should be noted that such doses could exceed the Tolerable Upper Intake Level (UL) for vitamin B_6.

Choline, an amine, is found naturally in a variety of foods and its RDA is grouped with the B vitamins. Choline is involved in the formation of acetylcholine, a neurotransmitter whose reduction in the nervous system may be theorized to be a contributing factor to the development of fatigue. Because plasma choline levels have been reported to be significantly reduced following marathon running, choline supplementation has been theorized to prevent fatigue. Research has shown that choline supplementation will increase blood choline levels at rest and during prolonged exercise, and some preliminary field and laboratory research has suggested increased plasma choline levels are associated with a significantly decreased time to run 20 miles. However, other well-controlled laboratory research has revealed that choline supplementation, although increasing plasma choline levels, exerted no effect on either brief, high-intensity anaerobic cycling tests or more prolonged aerobic exercise tasks. For example, choline supplementation, although increasing plasma free choline in marathon runners, had no effect on predicted or actual marathon time.

Multivitamin or Minerals

Multivitamin or mineral supplements are unnecessary for athletes or other physically active individuals who are on a well-balanced diet with adequate calories. For example, several studies have provided Multivitamin or mineral supplements over prolonged periods and reported no significant effects on both laboratory and sport-specific tests of physical performance. In one of the most comprehensive studies, Telford and others evaluated the effect of long term (7–8 months) vitamin/mineral supplementation (100 to 5,000 times the RDA) on exercise performance of nationally ranked athletes in training at the Australian Institute of Sport. The athletes were tested on a variety of sport-specific tasks as well as common tests of strength, anaerobic power, and aerobic endurance. They reported no significant effect of the supplementation protocol on any measure of physical performance when compared to athletes whose vitamin and mineral RDA were met by normal dietary intake.

Antioxidants

Antioxidant vitamins include vitamins C, E and beta-carotene, while coenzyme Q_{10} (CoQ_{10}) is a lipid with vitamin characteristics. Antioxidant vitamins have been studied individually and collectively for their potential to enhance exercise performance or to prevent exercise-induced muscle tissue damage.

Antioxidants and Exercise Performance

Vitamin C supplementation has been shown to improve physical performance in vitamin C-deficient subjects, but several major reviews support the general conclusion that vitamin C supplementation does not enhance physical performance in well-nourished individuals.

Vitamin E has been shown to enhance oxygen utilization during exercise at altitude, but does not appear to be an effective ergogenic under sea level conditions. A contemporary review indicated that although vitamin E supplementation may increase tissue or serum vitamin E concentration, most evidence suggests there is no discernable effect on training, performance, or rate of post-exercise recovery in either recreational or elite athletes. CoQ_{10}, also known as ubiquinone, is an antioxidant and may improve oxygen uptake in the mitochondria of the heart, and has been used therapeutically for the treatment of cardiovascular disease. Theoretically, improved oxygen usage in the heart and skeletal muscles could improve aerobic endurance performance. Only limited data are available, but these studies have shown that CoQ_{10} supplementation to healthy young or older subjects did not influence lipid peroxidation, heart rate, maximal oxygen uptake, anaerobic threshold, or cycling endurance performance. One study reported that CoQ_{10} supplementation was associated with muscle tissue damage and actually impaired cycling performance compared to the placebo treatment. Overall, there is limited evidence that dietary supplementation with antioxidants improves human performance.

Antioxidants and Muscle Tissue Damage

Strenuous exercise may generate reactive oxygen species (ROS) to a level to overwhelm tissue antioxidant defense systems. The result is oxidative stress, and one possible outcome is oxidative damage to muscle tissues. Preventing muscle tissue damage during exercise training may help optimize the training effect and eventual competitive sports performance. Numerous studies have evaluated the potential of antioxidant vitamin supplementation to prevent exercise-induced muscle tissue damage, and several extensive reviews have evaluated the available literature. However, the viewpoints of the reviewers vary somewhat.

Several reviewers conclude that antioxidant vitamin supplementation does not appear to prevent exercise-induced muscle tissue damage. Goldfarb concluded that research findings, mostly conducted with vitamin C, vitamin E, and beta carotene, have indicated that clear evidence for their prophylactic effect on various types of muscle damage following exercise is lacking. Other reviews have indicated that although animal studies have shown some promising effects of antioxidant supplementation to lessen exercise-induced oxidative stress damage, studies with humans are less convincing.

Contrarily, Dekkers and others concluded that dietary supplementation with antioxidant vitamins has favorable effects on lipid peroxidation and exercise-induced muscle damage and recommend vitamin supplementation to individuals performing regular heavy exercise. Evans noted that several antioxidants, including vitamin C and especially vitamin E, have been shown to decrease the exercise-induced increase in the rate of lipid peroxidation, which could help prevent muscle tissue damage. Other researchers are convinced that vitamin E contributes to preventing exercise-induced lipid peroxidation and possible muscle tissue damage, and recommend that athletes supplement with 100–200 milligrams of vitamin E daily to help prevent exercise-induced oxidative damage. Jiindicates that the delicate balance between pro-oxidants and antioxidants suggests that supplementation of antioxidants may be desirable for physically active individuals under certain physiological conditions by providing a larger protective margin. In particular, Jinotes that the aging process lessens the exercise training-induced improvement in natural antioxidant enzymes and suggests exercise training in older athletes might be assisted with antioxidant supplementation in attempts to optimize antioxidant defense.

Sacheck and Blumbergconcluded that the use of dietary antioxidants like vitamin E to reduce exercise-induced muscle injury have met with mixed success, which seems to be the prevailing viewpoint. All reviewers indicate more research is needed to address this issue and to provide guidelines for recommendations to athletes.

Vitamin and Mineral Supplements

Vitamin, mineral and trace element supplements are beneficial if they supply a nutrient that is deficient in the diet. That is, when dietary intake is lower than the amount needed to provide maximum benefit as judged from all biological perspectives. It is difficult to accurately define nutrient "adequacy" in competitive athletes, for several reasons. First, requirements for vitamins and minerals vary: metabolic, environmental, and genetic factors can influence individual nutrient requirements. Second, physical activity and physical fitness are complex, involving multiple diverse components that are difficult to accurately and reliably measure. Third, a nutrient supplement that could improve performance by as little as 2–3% could provide a competitive edge; for example, reducing a 1500 m runner's time of 3 min 45 s by 6 s. In order to detect such small changes an intervention requires randomized, placebo-controlled, double-blind studies designed to maximize statistical power. Inadequately designed studies may produce results that are unreliable and increase the likelihood a true effect will be missed. For these reasons, for many of the vitamins and minerals, it is difficult to argue forcefully for or against supplementation, and many competitive athletes choose to supplement.

However, there is general agreement that moderate physical activity does not adversely affect micronutrient status when diets provide recommended amounts of the vitamins, minerals and trace elements. Moreover, most studies have found that, because athletes tend to consume higher amounts of food to balance increased energy needs, their diets contain the recommended dietary allowance (RDA) of the essential micronutrients. Exceptions to this general rule are athletes on weight-loss diets, those with restrictive diets, vegetarians, and those with eating disorders – dietary patterns often found in sports that promote unrealistically low body fat. In such cases, a broad-spectrum vitamin/mineral supplement at the level of the RDA may be beneficial.

Vitamin E

Exercise increases the production of oxygen free radicals. Free radicals in muscle during or after exercise can arise from: 1) the mitochondrial respiratory chain; 2) the capillary endothelium; and 3) inflammatory cells mobilized because of muscle damage. If production overwhelms the cellular antioxidant defense system, membrane lipid peroxidation occurs. This can disrupt the membrane bilayer and impair enzyme and receptor function. Strenuous exercise, particularly in unconditioned individuals, can produce oxidative damage and muscle injury. In vivo and in vitro and human studies have reported free radical generation during and after exercise. Prolonged submaximal exercise increases whole-body and skeletal muscle lipid peroxidation byproducts.

Multiple enzymatic and nonenzymatic cellular antioxidant defense systems reduce damage to membranes and other cell structures from free radicals, and aerobic exercise training strengthens these antioxidant defenses. Membrane-bound vitamin E is abundant in the inner mitochondria, the site of the electron transport system. In rats, acute submaximal exercise reduces vitamin E concentrations in skeletal muscle and increases requirements for the vitamin. In exercised rats, vitamin E deficiency increases susceptibility to oxidative damage of lysosomal membranes, and is associated with earlier exhaustion and a ~40% decline in endurance capacity.

Meydani et al. reported that vitamin E supplementation (800 mg all-rac-α-tocopherol·d^{-1} for 30 d) increased skeletal muscle α-tocopherol by 53%. Vitamin E supplementation in humans reduces oxidative stress, lipid peroxidation and muscle soreness after exercise in some, but not all studies. Dillard et al. gave subjects 1200 IU α-tocopherol·d^{-1} for 2 wk and found a significant reduction in expired pentane at rest and during exercise. Sumida et al. reported that vitamin E decreased exerciseinduced increases in circulating glutamic-oxaloacetic transaminase (aspartate transaminase), ß-glucuronidase, and rate of lipid peroxidation, but because there was no placebo group, the results may have been at least partially due to an adaptation effect. Supplementation with 800 mg α-tocopherol·d^{-1} for 48 d reduced exerciseinduced oxidative injury, as indicated by a sparing of muscle fatty acids, reduced muscle lipid-conjugated dienes and decreased excretion of urinary thiobarbituric acid adducts. Rokitzki et al. gave competitive cyclists 300 mg α-tocopherol·d^{-1} or placebo for 5 months and then tested their response to strenuous exercise. In the treatment group, the increase in serum malondialdehyde (MDA) and creatine kinase (an intramuscular protein released if membranes are damaged) was significantly reduced compared to placebo. In subjects given 300 mg vitamin E·d^{-1} for 6 wk or placebo, the activity of muscle enzymes (e.g., creatine kinase and lactate dehydrogenase) in blood after strenuous exercise were similar. Francis and Hoobler gave subjects 600 mg vitamin E·d^{-1} for 2 d before and 2 d after strenuous eccentric exercise, but found that muscle soreness was not reduced by supplementation. Although vitamin E supplementation may enhance performance at high altitude, most well-controlled studies have not found an ergogenic effect of vitamin E supplementation, either on performance during standard exercise tests or cardiorespiratory fitness tests.

Vitamin C

Water-soluble vitamin C in the muscle cytosol can serve as an electron donor to vitamin E radicals generated in membranes during oxidative stress. In human subjects, supplementation with 400 mg ascorbic acid·d^{-1} for 3 wk increased blood ascorbic acid concentrations but did not significantly reduce plasma MDA after a bench-stepping exercise. However, using the same supplementation schedule and exercise protocol, Jakeman and Maxwell reported the ascorbic acid group showed reduced strength loss in the triceps surae after exercise and faster recovery, suggesting vitamin C supplementation reduced muscle damage. Delayed-onset muscle soreness may be an indicator of muscle damage induced by exercise. Staton gave men 200 mg ascorbic acid·d^{-1} or placebo for 30 d, and then had them perform sit-up exercises to induce soreness. When they repeated the exercise 24 h later, the supplemented group was able to perform significantly more sit-ups than the placebo group. Kaminski and Boal gave subjects 3 g ascorbic acid·d^{-1} or placebo for 3 d before eccentric exercise of the calf muscles. Compared to placebo, in half of the treated subjects there was a >33% reduction in soreness. However, well-controlled studies have found no benefit of ascorbic acid supplementation on either endurance or strength performance.

During aerobic training, adaptation to reduce oxidative damage may involve neutrophil monocyte accumulation in exercised muscle and secretion of cytokines, including IL-1, IL-1ß and tumor necrosis factor (TNF). In studies, IL-1 and TNF increase muscle proteolysis and release of amino acids. In humans, circulating IL-1 increases acutely after eccentric exercise, and downhill running significantly increases IL-1ß in the vastus lateralis. Supplementation with vitamins C and E may improve adaptive response to training by modifying circulating and muscle cytokines. After muscle-damaging exercise, supplementation with 1 g ascorbic acid given together with 400 mg all-rac-α-tocopherol has a greater effect on stimulating IL-1ß and TNF-α than does each vitamin alone.

Iron

Dietary iron (Fe) intake is marginal or inadequate in many females who engage in regular physical exercise. Basal obligatory losses in adults are ~1 mg $Fe \cdot d^{-1}$ and must be replaced by absorbed Fe to maintain balance. In many athletes, poor food choice and energy restriction to reduce body mass contributes to negative Fe balance. The Fe density of a typical meat-containing Western diet is 6 mg Fe/1000 kcal. Heme Fe (from meat, fish and poultry) is an important dietary source as it is better absorbed (5–35%) than nonheme Fe (2–20%). Because of lower dietary Fe density and reduced Fe bioavailability from plant foods, vegetarian athletes are at greater risk for Fe deficiency.

Increased Fe turnover and Fe losses also contribute to negative Fe balance during aerobic training. Fe losses may be due to covert gastrointestinal blood loss, increased Fe losses in sweat and erythrocyte hemolysis within the foot due to impact during running. In Fe-depleted rats, trained had higher erythrocyte Fe turnover than did non-exercise-trained. In humans, Ehn et al. found increased erythrocyte turnover in athletes and demonstrated that whole-body loss of Fe occurred ~20% faster in female athletes than in non-athletes.

The prevalence of Fe-deficiency anemia (IDA) in adults in Western countries (both athletes and non-athletes) is ~5–6%. The prevalence is higher in younger female athletes, because of needs for growth, menstrual losses, and, for some, energy restriction. Fe depletion, indicated by a low serum ferritin concentration, is common among athletes, with estimates of 35–50% among male and female endurance athletes. The prevalence of IDA may be lower among elite athletes: Wijn et al. measured Fe status in selected top-level athletes and found only 2% of male and 2.5% of female athletes were Fe-deficient anemic.

Depletion of the body's Fe stores decreases hemoglobin concentration and reduces oxygen transport capacity. In addition, reduced levels of myoglobin, mitochondrial cytochromes and other Fe-containing proteins in muscle may further lower aerobic capacity. During Fe depletion, these biochemical and physiological changes in muscle presage the decrease in hemoglobin concentration. IDA impairs oxygen delivery to tissues and reduces VO_2max, performance and endurance. Increasing dietary Fe intake and Fe supplementation can improve performance. Less clear are the effects of Fe supplementation on the athletic performance of those without reduced hemoglobin concentrations but with Fe depletion as evidenced by low serum ferritin. Limited evidence suggests Fe deficiency without anemia in women may reduce VO_2max, and that supplementation may be beneficial. Dietary changes, such as daily consumption of a single meat-containing meal, may help prevent decreases in ferritin associated with exercise. Although ≥60 mg supplemental Fe per day is recommended for treatment of IDA, moderate-level supplementation (40 mg $Fe \cdot d^{-1}$ as ferrous sulfate) prevented a decrease in serum ferritin in competitive swimmers.

Magnesium

Magnesium (Mg), a cofactor in >300 enzymatic reactions in cells, plays a fundamental role in energy metabolism. Mg is essential to many reactions, including glycogen breakdown, fat oxidation, protein synthesis, and ATP synthesis, particularly important during physical activity. Mg also serves as a physiologic regulator of membrane stability and is important in neuromuscular and cardiovascular function.

Dietary Mg intakes of physically active individuals generally are satisfactory; most surveys have reported intakes $\geq 70\%$ of the DRI. Comparing Mg intakes among physically active and age-matched control subjects Fogelholm et al. found greater Mg intakes among athletes than controls. Similarly, dietary Mg intake was higher among Nordic skiers than in their age- and sex-matched, nontraining counterparts. These differences appeared to be due to the athletes' higher energy intake and the greater Mg density of their diet. Longitudinal dietary monitoring of competitive female swimmers during training also reported adequate dietary Mg intakes. These studies do not suggest that physical activity per se increases risk of insufficient Mg intake.

In response to acute bouts of exercise, there is substantial redistribution of Mg within body compartments, as well as increased losses of Mg. During exercise, Mg shifts from the plasma into red blood cells, and urinary excretion of Mg significantly increases. Sweat losses of Mg also contribute: men exercising for 8 h on ergocycles lost 15–18 mg Mg$\cdot$d^{-1} in sweat that accounted for 4–5% of daily Mg intake and 10–15% of total Mg excretion. Recently, Lukaski and Nielsen examined the effects of dietary Mg restriction on physiologic responses during submaximal exercise. Peak oxygen uptake, total and cumulative net oxygen uptake, and peak heart rate increased during submaximal work when dietary Mg was restricted, suggesting Mg depletion adversely affected cardiovascular function.

Mg supplementation trials in athletes have produced mixed results. A limitation to studies of Mg supplementation in athletes is the lack of a sensitive indicator of status. Serum Mg concentration, although commonly used to evaluate Mg status in surveys, is a relatively insensitive index of marginal Mg status. In an anecdotal report, low serum Mg in a female tennis player with muscle spasms associated with prolonged outdoor exercise resolved with Mg supplementation (500 mg$\cdot$d^{-1}). Brilla and Haley gave men participating in a 7-wk strength training program and matched for quadriceps strength either a placebo or Mg supplements to obtain a total daily Mg intake of 8 mg/kg body mass. Total daily Mg intakes were 507 and 250 mg$\cdot$d^{-1} for the men receiving the Mg supplement and placebo, respectively. Peak knee-extension torque increased more in the Mgsupplemented than in the placebo-treated men. Golf et al. gave competitive rowers a Mg supplement (360 mg$\cdot$d^{-1}) for 4 wk and reported lower serum lactate concentrations and ~10% lower oxygen uptake during controlled submaximal exercise. In another supplementation trial, female athletes with marginally low plasma Mg received 360 mg$\cdot$d^{-1} as Mg aspartate or placebo for 3 wk. Compared to placebo, the treated group had significantly reduced total serum creatine kinase and creatine kinase isoenzyme from skeletal muscle after training. Trained adults given 250 mg Mg$\cdot$d^{-1} showed improved cardiorespiratory function during a 30-min submaximal exercise test compared to placebo. However, in a placebo-controlled trial, Mg supplementation (250 mg$\cdot$d^{-1}) of men in a 12-wk program of mainly aerobic or a combination of aerobic and anaerobic activities did not increase peak oxygen uptake, affect urinary Mg loss, or improve performance. A review of 12 well-controlled studies of Mg supplementation in humans and exercise performance concluded that the evidence is equivocal, regardless of whether the performance outcome was strength, anaerobic, or aerobic. Overall, studies suggest Mg supplementation does not affect performance when serum Mg is within the range of normal values, but may improve performance when marginal or clinical Mg deficiency is present. Trained subjects appear to benefit less than untrained subjects, and there is a lack of research in physically active females who may be at the highest risk for Mg deficiency.

Bodybuilding Supplement

Bodybuilding supplements are dietary supplements commonly used by those involved in bodybuilding, weightlifting, mixed martial arts, and athletics for the purpose of facilitating an increase in lean body mass. The intent is to increase muscle, increase body weight, improve athletic performance, and for some sports, to simultaneously decrease percent body fat so as to create better muscle definition. Among the most widely used are high protein drinks, branched-chain amino acids (BCAA), glutamine, arginine, essential fatty acids, creatine, HMB, and weight loss products. Supplements are sold either as single ingredient preparations or in the form of "stacks" – proprietary blends of various supplements marketed as offering synergistic advantages. While many bodybuilding supplements are also consumed by the general public the frequency of use will differ when used specifically by bodybuilders. One meta-analysis concluded that – for athletes participating in resistance exercise training and consuming protein supplements for an average of 13 weeks – total protein intake up to 1.6 g/kg of body weight per day would result in an increase in strength and fat-free mass, but that higher intakes would not further contribute.

Mislabeling and Adulteration

While many of the claims are based on scientifically based physiological or biochemical processes, their use in bodybuilding parlance is often heavily colored by bodybuilding lore and industry marketing and as such may deviate considerably from traditional scientific usages of the terms. In addition, ingredients listed have been found at times to be different from the contents. In 2015, Consumer Reports reported unsafe levels of arsenic, cadmium, lead and mercury in several of the protein powders that were tested.

In the United States, the manufacturers of dietary supplements do not need to provide the Food and Drug Administration with evidence of product safety prior to marketing. As a result, the incidence of products adulterated with illegal ingredients has continued to rise. In 2013, one-third of the supplements tested were adulterated with unlisted steroids. More recently, the prevalence of designer steroids with unknown safety and pharmacological effects has increased.

In 2015 a CBC investigative report found that protein spiking (the addition of amino acid filler to manipulate analysis) was not uncommon; however, many of the companies involved challenged these claims.

Health Problems

The US FDA reports 50,000 health problems a year due to dietary supplements and these often involve bodybuilding supplements. For example, the "natural" best-seller Craze, 2012's "New Supplement of the Year", widely sold in stores such as Walmart and Amazon, was found to contain N,alpha-Diethylphenylethylamine, a methamphetamine analog. Other products by Matt Cahill have contained dangerous substances causing blindness or liver damage, and experts say that Cahill is emblematic for the whole industry.

Liver Damage

The incidence of liver damage from herbal and dietary supplements is about 16–20% of all supplement products causing injury, with the occurrence growing globally over the early 21st century. The most common liver injuries from weight loss and bodybuilding supplements involve hepatocellular damage with resulting jaundice, and the most common supplement ingredients attributed to these injuries are catechins from green tea, anabolic steroids, and the herbal extract, aegeline.

Lack of Effectiveness

In addition to being potentially harmful, some have argued that there is little evidence to indicate any benefit to using bodybuilding protein or amino acid supplements. "In view of the lack of compelling evidence to the contrary, no additional dietary protein is suggested for healthy adults undertaking resistance or endurance exercise". In dispute of this, one more recent meta-analysis concluded that for athletes participating in resistance exercise training and consuming protein supplements for an average of 13 weeks, total protein intake up to 1.6 g per kg body weight per day would result in an increase in strength and fat-free mass, i.e. muscle, but that higher intakes would not further contribute. The muscle mass increase was statistically significant but modest - averaging 0.3 for all trials and 1.0 to 2.0 kg, for protein intake ≥ 1.6 g/kg/day.

Protein

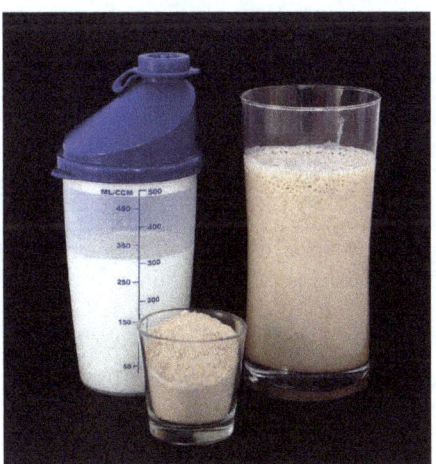

Protein shakes, made from protein powder (center) and
milk (left), are a common bodybuilding supplement.

Bodybuilders may supplement their diets with protein for reasons of convenience, lower cost (relative to meat and fish products), ease of preparation, and to avoid the concurrent consumption of carbohydrates and fats. Additionally, some argue that bodybuilders, by virtue of their unique training and goals, require higher-than-average quantities of protein to support maximal muscle growth. However, there is no scientific consensus for bodybuilders to consume more protein than the recommended dietary allowance. Protein supplements are sold in ready-to-drink shakes, bars, meal replacement products, bites, oats, gels and powders. Protein powders are the most popular and may have flavoring added for palatability. The powder is usually mixed with water, milk or fruit juice and is generally consumed immediately before and after exercising or in place of a meal. The sources of protein are as follows and differ in protein quality depending on their amino acid profile and digestibility:

- Whey protein contains high levels of all the essential amino acids and branched-chain amino acids. It also has the highest content of the amino acid cysteine, which aids in the biosynthesis of glutathione. For bodybuilders, whey protein provides amino acids used to aid in muscle recovery. Whey protein is derived from the process of making cheese from milk. There are three types of whey protein: whey concentrate, whey isolate, and whey hydrolysate. Whey concentrate is 29–89% protein by weight whereas whey isolate is 90%+ protein by weight. Whey hydrolysate is enzymatically predigested and therefore has the highest rate of digestion of all protein types.

- Casein protein (or milk protein) has glutamine, and casomorphin.

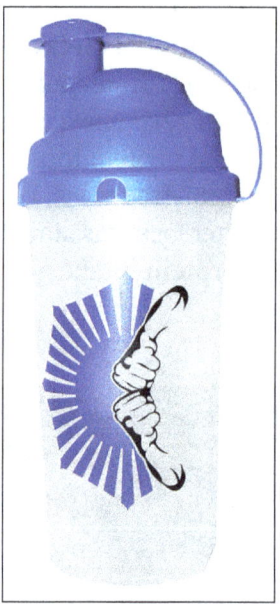

Shaker Bottle commonly used to mix supplements. Often has mesh or a metal whisk inside to breakdown lumps in the mixture.

Some nutritionists have suggested that higher calcium excretion may be due to a corresponding increase in protein-induced calcium absorption in the intestines.

Amino Acids

Some bodybuilders believe that amino acid supplements may benefit muscle development, but consumption of such supplements is unnecessary in a diet that already includes adequate protein intake.

Prohormones

Prohormones are precursors to hormones and are most typically sold to bodybuilders as a precursor to the natural hormone testosterone. This conversion requires naturally occurring enzymes in the body. Side effects are not uncommon, as prohormones can also convert further into DHT and estrogen. To deal with this, many supplements also have aromatase inhibitors and DHT blockers such as chrysin and 4-androstene-3,6,17-trione. To date most prohormone products have not been thoroughly studied, and the health effects of prolonged use are unknown. Although initially available over the counter, their purchase was made illegal without a prescription in the US in 2004, and they hold similar status in many other countries. They remain legal, however, in the United Kingdom and the wider European Union. Their use is prohibited by most sporting bodies.

Creatine

Creatine is an organic acid naturally occurring in the body that supplies energy to muscle cells for short bursts of energy (as required in lifting weights) via creatine phosphate replenishment of ATP. A number of scientific studies have shown that creatine can improve strength, energy, muscle mass, and recovery times. In addition, recent studies have also shown that creatine improves brain function. and reduces mental fatigue. Unlike steroids or other performance-enhancing drugs, creatine can be found naturally in many common foods such as herring, tuna, salmon, and beef.

Creatine increases what is known as cell volumization by drawing water into muscle cells, making them larger. This intracellular retention should not be confused with the common myth that creatine causes bloating (or intercellular water retention).

Creatine is sold in a variety of forms, including creatine monohydrate and creatine ethyl ester, amongst others. Though all types of creatine are sold for the same purposes, there are subtle differences between them, such as price and necessary dosage.

Some studies have suggested that consumption of creatine with protein and carbohydrates can have a greater effect than creatine combined with either protein or carbohydrates alone.

β-Hydroxy β-Methylbutyrate

When combined with an appropriate exercise program, dietary supplementation with β-hydroxy β-methylbutyrate (HMB) has been shown to dose-dependently augment gains in muscle hypertrophy (i.e., the size of a muscle), muscle strength, and lean body mass, reduce exercise-induced skeletal muscle damage,and expedite recovery from high-intensity exercise. HMB is believed to produce these effects by increasing muscle protein synthesis and decreasing muscle protein breakdown by various mechanisms, including activation of the mechanistic target of rapamycin (mTOR) and inhibition of the proteasome in skeletal muscles.

The inhibition of exercise-induced skeletal muscle damage by HMB is affected by the time that it is used relative to exercise. The greatest reduction in skeletal muscle damage from a single bout of exercise appears to occur when calcium HMB is ingested 1–2 hours prior to exercise.

Meal Replacement Products

Meal replacement products (MRPs) are either pre-packaged powdered drink mixes or edible bars designed to replace prepared meals. MRPs are generally high in protein, low in fat, have a low to moderate amount of carbohydrates, and contain a wide array of vitamins and minerals.

The majority of MRPs use whey protein, casein (often listed as calcium caseinate or micellar casein), soy protein, and egg albumin as protein sources. Carbohydrates are typically derived from maltodextrin, oat fiber, brown rice, and wheat flour. Some MRPs also contain flax oil powder as a source of essential fatty acids.

MRPs can also contain other ingredients, such as creatine monohydrate, glutamine peptides, L-glutamine, calcium alpha-ketoglutarate, additional amino acids, lactoferrin, conjugated linoleic acid, and medium-chain triglycerides.

A sub-class of MRPs is colloquially known as "weight gainers", which are meal replacement products with a higher carbohydrate:protein ratio. Whereas a MRP will typically have a 0.25-2:1 carbohydrate:protein ratio, a weight gainer might have a ratio in the order of 3-5:1.

Thermogenic Products

A thermogenic is a broad term for any supplement that the manufacturer claims will cause thermogenesis, resulting in increased body temperature, increased metabolic rate, and consequently an increased rate in the burning of body fat and weight loss. Until 2004 almost every product found in this supplement category comprised the "ECA stack": ephedrine, caffeine and aspirin. However, on February 6, 2004 the Food and Drug Administration (FDA) banned the sale of ephedra and its alkaloid, ephedrine, for use in weight loss formulas. Several manufacturers replaced the ephedra component of the "ECA" stack with bitter orange or citrus aurantium (containing synephrine) instead of the ephedrine.

Whey Protein

Whey protein is a mixture of proteins isolated from whey, the liquid material created as a by-product of cheese production. The proteins consist of α-lactalbumin, β-lactoglobulin, serum albumin and immunoglobulins. Whey protein is commonly marketed as a dietary supplement, and various health claims have been attributed to it.

Production of Whey

Whey is left over when milk is coagulated during the process of cheese production, and contains everything that is soluble from milk after the pH is dropped to 4.6 during the coagulation process. It is a 5% solution of lactose in water with lactalbumin and some lipid content. Processing can be done by simple drying, or the relative protein content can be increased by removing the lactose, lipids and other non-protein materials. For example, spray drying after membrane filtration separates the proteins from whey.

Whey can be denatured by heat. High heat (such as the sustained high temperatures above 72 °C associated with the pasteurization process) denatures whey proteins. While native whey protein does not aggregate upon renneting or acidification of milk, denaturing the whey protein triggers hydrophobic interactions with other proteins, and the formation of a protein gel.

Composition

The protein in cow's milk is 20% whey and 80% casein. The protein in human milk is 60% whey and 40% casein. The protein fraction in whey constitutes approximately 10% of the total dry solids in whey. This protein is typically a mixture of beta-lactoglobulin (~65%), alpha-lactalbumin (~25%), bovine serum albumin (~8%), and immunoglobulins. These are soluble in their native forms, independent of pH.

Major Forms and Uses

Commercially produced whey protein from cow's milk typically comes in four major forms:

- Concentrates (WPC) have typically a low (but still significant) level of fat and cholesterol but, in general, compared to the other forms of whey protein, they are higher in carbohydrates in the form of lactose — they are 29%–89% protein by weight.

- Isolates (WPI) are processed to remove the fat and lactose — they are 90%+ protein by weight. Like whey protein concentrates, whey protein isolates are mild to slightly milky in taste.

- Hydrolysates (WPH) are whey proteins that are predigested and partially hydrolyzed for the purpose of easier metabolizing, but their cost is generally higher. Highly hydrolysed whey may be less allergenic than other forms of whey.

- Native whey protein is extracted from skim milk, not a byproduct of cheese production, and produced as a concentrate and isolate.

There is evidence that whey protein is better absorbed than casein or soy protein.

Whey protein is commonly marketed as a dietary supplement, typically sold in powdered form for mixing into beverages. The products have varying proportions of the major forms above, and are promoted with various health claims. In 2010 a panel of the European Food Safety Authority (EFSA) examined proposed health claims made for whey protein: satiety, weight loss, reduced body fat, increased muscle, increased strength, increased endurance and faster recovery after exercising. The EFSA concluded that the provided literature did not adequately support the proposed claims.

Although whey proteins are responsible for some milk allergies, the major allergens in milk are the caseins.

Creatine Supplements

Creatine is a nitrogenous organic acid that helps supply energy to cells throughout the body, particularly muscle cells.

It occurs naturally in red meat and fish, it is made by the body, and it can also be obtained from supplements.

Supplements are used by athletes to improve their performance, by older adults to increase muscle mass, and to treat problems that result when a body cannot metabolize creatine fully.

Some evidence suggests that it might prevent skin aging, treat muscle diseases, help people with multiple sclerosis (MS) to exercise, enhance cognitive ability, and more. Additional evidence is needed to confirm these uses.

Creatine is formed of three amino acids: L-arginine, glycine, and L-methionine. It makes up about 1 percent of the total volume of human blood.

Around 95 percent of creatine in the human body is stored in skeletal muscle, and 5 percent is in the brain.

Between 1.5 and 2 percent of the body's creatine store is converted for use each day by the liver, the kidneys, and the pancreas.

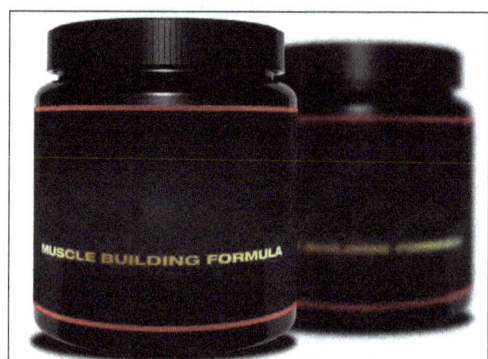

Creatine is a common ingredient muscle-building supplements and sports drinks.

It is transported through the blood and used by parts of the body that have high energy demands, such as skeletal muscle and the brain.

Different forms of creatine are used in supplements, including creatine monohydrate and creatine nitrate.

No creatine supplement has yet been approved for use by the United States (U.S.) Food and Drug Administration (FDA). There are dangers associated with use of unrestricted supplements.

Source and Needs

A person needs between 1 and 3 grams (g) of creatine a day. Around half of this comes from the diet, and the rest is synthesized by the body. Food sources include red meat and fish. One pound of raw beef or salmon provides 1 to 2 grams (g) of creatine.

Creatine can supply energy to parts of the body where it is needed. Athletes use supplements to increase energy production, improve athletic performance, and to allow them to train harder.

According to the International Society of Sports Nutrition (ISSN), larger athletes who train intensely "may need to consume between 5 and 10 g of creatine a day" to maintain their stores.

People who cannot synthesize creatine because of a health condition may need to take 10 to 30 g a day to avoid health problems.

Uses

Creatine is one of the most popular supplements, especially among men who participate in ice hockey, football, baseball, lacrosse, and wrestling.

It is also the most common supplement found in sports nutrition supplements, including sports drinks.

There are claims for a number of uses, some of which are supported by research evidence.

Improving Athletic Performance

Athletes commonly use creatine supplements, because there is some evidence that they are effective in high-intensity training.

The idea is that creatine allows the body to produce more energy. With more energy, athletes can work harder and achieve more.

For some participants in some kinds of exercise, boosting the body's creatine pool appears to enhance performance.

In 2003, a meta-analysis concluded that creatine "may improve performance involving short periods of extremely powerful activity, especially during repeated bouts."

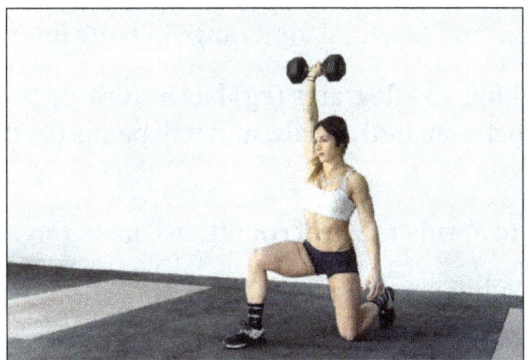
Creatine is popular with athletes.

The researchers added that not all studies had reported the same benefits.

A review concluded that creatine:

- Boosts the effects of resistance training on strength and body mass.

- Increases the quality and benefits of high-intensity intermittent speed training.

- Improves endurance performance in aerobic exercise activities that last more than 150 seconds.

- May improve strength, power, fat-free mass, daily living performance and neurological function.

It seems to benefit athletes participating in anaerobic exercise, but not in aerobic activity.

It appears to be useful in short-duration, high-intensity, intermittent exercises, but not necessarily in other types of exercise.

However, a study published in 2017 found that creatine supplementation did not boost fitness or performance in 17 young female athletes who used it for 4 weeks.

Increased Body Mass

Increased creatine content in muscles has been associated with greater body mass.

However, creatine does not build muscle. The increase in body mass occurs because creatine causes the muscles to hold water.

It is also possible that muscle mass builds as a result of working harder during exercise.

Repairing Damage after Injury

Research suggests that creatine supplements may help prevent muscle damage and enhance the recovery process after an athlete has experienced an injury.

Creatine may also have an antioxidant effect after an intense session of resistance training, and it may help reduce cramping. It may have a role in rehabilitation for brain and other injuries.

Creatine and Deficiency Syndromes

Creatine is a natural substance and essential for a range of body functions.

An average young male weighing 70 kilograms (kg) has a store, or pool, of creatine of around 120 to 140 g. The amount varies between individuals, and it depends partly on a person's muscle mass and their muscle fiber type.

Creatine deficiency is linked to a wide range of conditions, including, but not limited to:

- Chronic Obstructive Pulmonary Disease (Copd).
- Congestive heart failure (CHF).
- Depression.
- Diabetes.
- Multiple Sclerosis (Ms).
- Muscle atrophy.
- Parkinson's disease.
- Fibromyalgia.
- Osteoarthritis.

Oral creatine supplements may relieve these conditions, but there is not yet enough evidence to prove that this is an effective treatment for most of them.

Supplements are also taken to increase creatine in the brain. This can help relieve seizures, symptoms of autism, and movement disorders.

Taking creatine supplements for up to 8 years has been shown to improve attention, language and academic performance in some children. However, it does not affect everyone in the same way.

While creatine occurs naturally in the body, creatine supplements are not a natural substance. Anyone considering using these or other supplements should do so only after researching the company that provides them.

Soy Protein

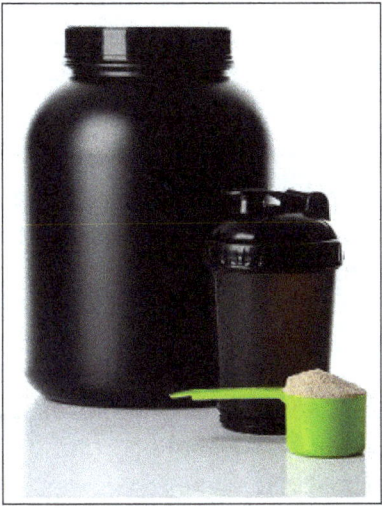

Soy is the least commonly used protein among athletes. It is probably a common Soy Protein 1 Canadian Academy of Sports Nutrition caasnsupplement among vegetarians. Soy protein is a complete protein that comes from soybean. Soybean is considered a legume.

Digestibility and Absorption

Soy protein has the biologic value (BV) of 74, which is lower than those of whey (with BV over 100) and casein (with BV of 77). Though soy is a compete protein and has all the essential amino acids, it is considered a low quality protein. However, soy protein has some health advantages compared to whey and casein proteins.

Soy protein is digested by the same enzymes that break down whey and casein. The digestibility of soy protein is about 95%, while it is 65% for soybeans. The absorption of soy protein is faster than that of casein protein and slower than that of whey protein.

Compositions of Soy

Amino acid compositions of soy are different than those of whey, casein, and egg proteins. Compared to whey, soy is higher in glutamine.

A unique compound in soy protein is phytoestrogens. They are phytonutrients with many health benefits. The estrogenic effects of soy are more prominent in female athletes than male athletes.

The main phytoestrogens in soy protein are isoflavones, of which genistein and daidzein are the major ones. Isoflavones are important in bone health.

Isoflavones in Soy Products	
Soy products	Isoflavones (mg per one gram of the product)
Soy flour	2.6
Fermented soybean	1.3
Fried soybean curd	0.7
Cooked soybean	0.6
Soy protein powder	0.5
Soybean curd	0.5
Soy milk	0.4
Soybean paste	0.4
Soy sauce	0.015

Another distinctive ingredient of soy protein is "*lunasin*". It is a soy dipeptide that can be found in rye, barley, and wheat as well. It is claimed that lunasin has anti – inflammatory and anti – cancer activities, particularly against leukemia.

Indications of using Soy Protein

Soy protein has many health benefits especially in women, as it contains phytoestrogens.

Athletic Indications of Soy Protein

Female athletes may benefit from soy protein more than male athletes. Soy protein could be beneficial in the following conditions:

- Female Athlete Triad Syndrome (FATS).

- Vegetarian and vegan athletes.

- Female athletes with any estrogen – sensitive cancers.

- Elderly female gym – goers with Osteoporosis.

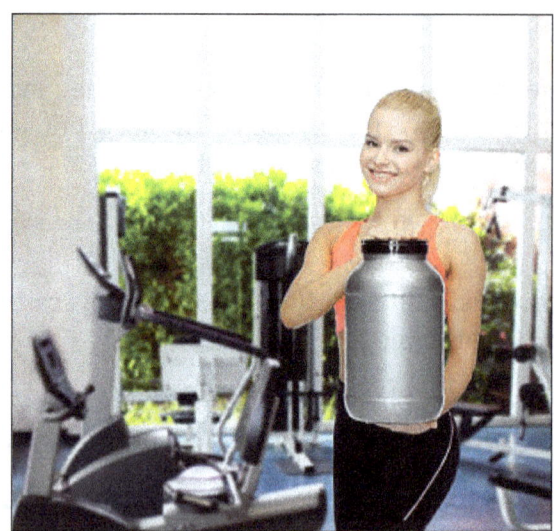

Non-athletic Indications of Soy Protein

Soy protein may be useful in the following conditions:

- High levels of LDL cholesterol and triglyceride.

- Menopause.

- Osteoporosis.

- Estrogen – sensitive cancers.

- Diabetes.

- Vegetarians and vegans.

- Infants with lactase deficiency (as soy – based formulas).

- Infants with galactosemia (as soy – based formulas).

Taking Soy Protein

Soy protein is available in different formulations in the market, providing 20 – 25 grams of soy protein per serving. The ideal daily intake of soy protein has not been established yet, and it depends on the total daily requirement of protein and health status.

- Athletes: 30 – 50 grams a day upon wake up or after exercise.

- Athletes with Female Athlete Triad Syndrome: 50 – 70 grams a day upon wake up or after exercise.

- Osteoporosis: 40 grams a day of soy protein with 2 mg of isoflavones per one gram of powder.

- Menopause: 30 – 60 grams a day of soy protein with 40 – 60 mg of isoflavones.

- Vegetarians and vegans: 30 – 60 grams a day.

- High LDL cholesterol: 30 – 60 grams a day.

- Diabetes: 30 grams a day.

Interactions and Cautions

Soy protein and fermented soy products have interactions with the following medications:

- MAOIs (monoamine oxidase inhibitors): These medications are used to treat depression and anxiety disorders. Fermented soy products contain tyramine. It is an amino acid that involves in regulating blood pressure and is needed to be metabolized by monoamine oxidase. MAOIs inhibit the breakdown of tyramine, leading to sudden increase in blood pressure. These medications include:

  - Isocarboxazid (Marplan).

  - Phenelzine (Nardi).

- Selegiline (Emsam).
- Tranylcypromine (Parnate).

- Antibiotics: They decrease the effectiveness of soy protein.
- Probiotics: They increase the effectiveness of soy.
- Warfarin: Soy may decrease the effectiveness of this medication.
- Birth control pills: Soy may decrease the effectiveness of these pills.
- Tamoxifen: Soy may decrease the effectiveness of this medication.
- Thyroid medications: Soy may interfere with the absorption of these medications.

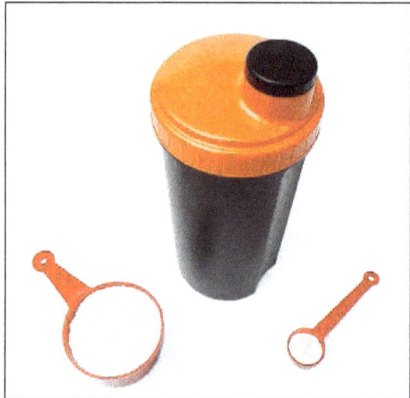

Soy protein should be used with extreme caution in the following medical conditions:

- Liver diseases.
- Kidney diseases.
- Chronic pancreatitis.
- Hartnup syndrome.
- Cystinuria.

Soy protein should be avoided in the following medical conditions:

- Acute renal failure.
- Hepatic encephalopathy.
- Diabetic nephropathy.
- Rhabdomyolysis.
- Low function thyroid.

Some studies indicate that isoflavones in soy may inhibit TPO (thyroid peroxidase) and interfere with normal function of the thyroid. The amount of soy isoflavones that could affect the function of thyroid gland is about 30 mg per day.

- Children with congenital hypothyroidism. They should not be feed by soy – based formulas.

- Goiter.

Side Effects

Allergic reactions to soy protein are less common than to whey and casein proteins. Some other reported side effects of soy protein are nausea, constipation, sleepiness, and fatigue.

Performance-enhancing Substance

Performance-enhancing substances, also known as performance-enhancing drugs (PED), are substances that are used to improve any form of activity performance in humans. A well-known example involves doping in sport, where banned physical performance–enhancing drugs are used by athletes and bodybuilders. Athletic performance-enhancing substances are sometimes referred to as ergogenic aids. Cognitive performance-enhancing drugs, commonly called nootropics, are sometimes used by students to improve academic performance. Performance-enhancing substances are also used by military personnel to enhance combat performance.

The use of performance-enhancing drugs spans the categories of legitimate use and substance abuse.

The classifications of substances as performance-enhancing substances are not entirely clear-cut and objective. As in other types of categorization, certain prototype performance enhancers are universally classified as such (like anabolic steroids), whereas other substances (like vitamins and protein supplements) are virtually never classified as performance enhancers despite their effects on performance. As is usual with categorization, there are borderline cases; caffeine, for example, is considered a performance enhancer by some but not others.

Types

The phrase has been used to refer to several distinct classes of drugs:

- Anabolic drugs build up muscle; examples include: steroids, hormones, most notably human growth hormone, as well as some of their prodrugs, selective androgen receptor modulators, and beta-2 agonists.

- Stimulants improve focus and alertness. Low (therapeutic) doses of dopaminergic stimulants (e.g., reuptake inhibitors and releasing agents) also promote cognitive and athletic performance, as nootropics and ergogenic aids respectively, by improving muscle strength and endurance while decreasing reaction time and fatigue; some examples of athletic performance-enhancing stimulants are caffeine, ephedrine, methylphenidate, and amphetamine.

- Ergogenic aids, or athletic performance-enhancing substances, include a number of drugs with various effects on physical performance. Drugs such as amphetamine and methylphenidate increase power output at constant levels of perceived exertion and delay the onset of fatigue, among other athletic-performance-enhancing effects; bupropion also increases power output at constant levels of perceived exertion, but only during short term use. Creatine, a nutritional supplement that is commonly used by athletes, increases high-intensity exercise capacity.

- Human biomolecules – creatine and β-hydroxy β-methylbutyrate are naturally occurring compounds in humans that have well-established ergogenic effects and effects on body composition when supplemented.

- Adaptogens are plants that support health through nonspecific effects, neutralize various environmental and physical stressors while being relatively safe and free of side effects. As of 2008, the position of the European Medicines Agency was that "The principle of an adaptogenic action needs further clarification and studies in the pre-clinical and clinical area. As such, the term is not accepted in pharmacological and clinical terminology that is commonly used in the EU."

- Nootropics, or "cognition enhancers", benefit overall cognition by improving memory (e.g., increasing working memory capacity or updating) or other aspects of cognitive control (e.g., inhibitory control, attentional control, attention span, etc.).

- Painkillers allow performance beyond the usual pain threshold. Some painkillers raise blood pressure, increasing oxygen supply to muscle cells. Painkillers used by athletes range from common over-the-counter medicines such as NSAIDs (such as ibuprofen) to powerful prescription narcotics.

- Sedatives and anxiolytics are sometimes used in sports like archery which require steady hands and accurate aim, and also to overcome excessive nervousness or discomfort. Diazepam and propranolol are common examples; ethanol and cannabis are also used occasionally.

- Blood boosters (blood doping agents) increase the oxygen-carrying capacity of blood beyond the individual's natural capacity. They are used in endurance sports like long-distance running, cycling, and Nordic skiing. Recombinant human erythropoietin (rhEPO) is one of the most widely known drugs in this class.

- Gene doping agents are a relatively recently described class of athletic performance-enhancing substances. These drug therapies, which involve viral vector-mediated gene transfer.

Usage in Sport

In sports, the phrase performance-enhancing drugs is popularly used in reference to anabolic steroids or their precursors (hence the colloquial term "steroids"); anti-doping organizations apply the term broadly. There are agencies such as WADA and USADA that try to prevent athletes from using these drugs by performing drug tests. WADA was founded on November 10, 1999 by Dick Pound. The World Anti-doping Agency focuses on establishing and enforcing rules and codes for all sports around the world. Their goal is to make all sports played fairly between all athletes in a doping free organization with the power to prevent athletes from using any form of performance-enhancing drugs. USADA started October 1, 2000 as non-profit and was composed of nine members. Five of which were former Olympic athletes with the other four elected from independent companies. This is the United States Anti-doping Agency and have the ability to test athletes across the nation. Steroids and performance-enhancing drugs are used across all sports organizations around the world.

Ergolytic Agents

Ergolytic is the opposite of ergogenic. The term ergolytic is used to refer to an agent, device, or factor that impairs athletic performance rather than enhances it. This impairment can be the result of physiological or psychological factors. Some common ergolytic agents are alcohol, tobacco (including smokeless), and marijuana.

Some supplements or other products that are thought to be ergogenic for one aspect of performance may be ergolytic for other aspects of performance. For instance, although creatine is thought, with good evidence, to enhance short-term anaerobic metabolism, it has been suggested that this increase could produce more lactate and subject an athlete to more lactic acidosis.

Diet can be potentially ergolytic. A caloric excess resulting in weight gain, for instance, could impair performance for endurance athletes and relative strength athletes. A diet without adequate carbohydrate could impair performance for an endurance athlete, as well.

Beta Blockers

Beta blockers are used as an ergogenic aid in archery and shooting, but will likely impair performance, perhaps greatly, in endurance and strength athletes. These drugs, such as Inderal (propranalol) and Tenormin (atenalo), are used to treat high blood pressure. These drugs attenuate the heart rate and blood pressure response to exercise and also decrease tidal volume, increasing respiratory rate. They can speed time to exhaustion and impair the body's ability to regulate temperature. It is possible that some eye drops used to treat glaucoma, such as timilol, another beta blocker, may be absorbed into the body and worsen performance.

Calcium Channel Blockers

Calcium channel blockers are blood pressure and angina medications such as Diltiazem and Verapamil. They decrease heart rate response to exercise and may decrease myocardial contractility.

Alpha blockers are other blood pressure medications that are potentially ergolytic.

Antihistamines

Anthihistamines are commonly used over-the-counter remedies for cold and allergy symptoms such as diphenhydramine, chlorpheniramine, and loratadine. They can cause drowsiness, which would certainly impair performance. They can also decrease psychomotor performance.

Antacids

Other common over-the-counter medicines may also be ergolytic. Among them are antacids such as Tagamet (cimitidene), which has been found to be anti-androgenic to a small number of men, causing breast enlargement and inhibited sexual function. Interference with testosterone could reduce muscle mass and interfere with performance.

Caffeine

Caffeine is one of the most widely consumed drugs in the world, readily available in coffee, tea, and soft drinks, is also one of the most wildly popular ergogenic aids, with proven benefits to performance. However, it can also become an ergolytic for several reasons.

People who are not used to caffeine or consume it in very large doses may experience nervousness, tremors, restlessness, insomnia, headache, and gastrointestinal problems. Disrupted sleep patterns can obviously impair performance. Since it acts as a diuretic, it may put athletes at risk for dehydration in hot environments. Also, caffeine is physically addictive, and abrupt cessation of use can cause severe headache (caffeine headache), fatigue, irritability and gastrointestinal distress.

Inosine

Inosine is a purine based nucleotide which is a structural component of ATP. It is obtained in the diet or produced endogenously in the body. It has been marketed as a dietary supplement and claimed by manufacturers to increase ATP stores, and so increase muscle strength and training performance. It has also been said to increase oxygen delivery to the cells to improve endurance. This is based on the role that inosine plays in the formation of 2-3-diphosphoglycerate, a substance in erythrocytes that facilitates the release of oxygen to the tissues. Other benefits have also been postulated. No studies have provided support for these claims or theories and one study found an ergolytic effect, where time to fatigue was decreased. Perhaps more importantly, it increases uric acid levels to amounts associated with gouty arthritis, which cause joint pain, particularly in the knee and foot.

References

- Sports-drinks: diabetes.co.uk, Retrieved 29 June, 2019, Retrieved 14 July, 2019

- Ronald Hamowy (2007), Government and public health in America (illustrated ed.), Edward Elgar Publishing, pp. 140–141, ISBN 978-1-84542-911-9

- Sports-drinks, fuelling-recovery, factsheets: sportsdietitians.com.au, Retrieved 18 April, 2019

- Fred W. Sauceman (1 March 2009). The Place Setting: Timeless Tastes of the Mountain South, from Bright Hope to Frog Level. Mercer University Press. Pp. 89–. ISBN 978-0-88146-140-4

- What-drinks-are-diet-have-electrolytes: livestrong.com, Retrieved 21 July, 2019

- Purpose-recovery-drink: sfgate.com, Retrieved 13 July, 2019

- Food-and-drinks-for-sport, eat-well, live-well: nhs.uk, Retrieved 24 March, 2019

- Schwarb, John (January 3, 2003). "Forget carb-filled bars, runners gaga for goo". St. Petersburg Times. St. Petersburg, Florida. Retrieved January 13, 2014

4

Adverse Effects of Supplements

Supplements affect the health of the athletes adversely. It can cause bloating, muscle cramps, nausea, stroke, heart diseases, liver damage, high cholesterol, high blood pressure, infertility, etc. This chapter closely examines these adverse effects of supplements to provide an extensive understanding of the subject.

Supplements and their Risks

'Supplement' is an overarching name for vitamins, minerals, herbal remedies, traditional Asian remedies, amino acids and other substances to be taken orally. They may also be referred to as dietary, food or nutritional supplements or ergogenic aids (supplements purported to improve athletic performance) and are typically sold in the form of tablets, capsules, soft gels, liquids, powders, and bars. Supplements are not required to exhibit efficacy before marketing, nor are they subject to prior approval unless they are genetically modified or claimed to be new. Medicinal claims on packaging or in an advertisement for a supplement, however, are prohibited.

Widespread debate has accompanied the introduction of new legislation on the use of dietary supplements. Some thirty thousand supplements are commercially-available in the USA with approximately half of the adult female population being regular users, with possible adverse effects of unregulated supplement use on health and disease outcomes being of particular interest.

Supplement use in Sport

For some 50 years, competitive sports have operated under strict regulation, and adherence to the ever-growing list of prohibited substances is expected from all high performing athletes at all times. Gaining competitive advantage, however, is more important than ever. Personal satisfaction as well as the athletes' livelihoods and their organisations' prosperity depend on success. Athletes naturally turn to supplements hoping to find herbs, vitamins or minerals that provide the desired competitive edge.

Worldwide supplement use among athletes, on average, ranges between 40 and 60 percent. Nutri-tional supplements are typically used for their actual or anecdotal physiological effects in increasing performance and endurance, health maintenance or preventing injuries, and the extent and amount of ergogenic 'drugs' and supplements used by athletes shows a growing trend. Research linking supplement use to involvement in physical activity and previous studies on decision making patterns among these groups has focused on user subgroup classifications. While this enables an understanding of the gross difference in the patterns of use between groups of users, it fails to give an explanation for why those differences might occur. One key understudied aspect is a poten-tial mismatch between the decision making and execution in practice.

Numerous factors can be involved in athletes' decisions to use supplements including desired end points such as increasing strength, endurance, training duration and overcoming injury as well as avoid-ing sickness and compensating for poor diet. Unfortunately, lack of knowledge and misconceptions regarding supplements within athlete populations have been documented for more than a decade. Recent research also shows that athletes are willing to take supplements based on personal recommen-dation without gathering reliable information about the substances, often obtaining them directly from retailers and internet sites. Adolescents are more willing to take supplements obediently if they are informed by their parents/guardians, as opposed to by coaches or resulting from published research.

Conflicting reports on knowledge levels within health care professions demonstrate a wide varia-tion in practice. In one study, physicians and medical students were tested to determine the level of their knowledge regarding efficacy and toxicity, and drug interactions with herbal remedies, and it was found that the mean test scores were only slightly higher than scores obtained from random guessing. On the contrary, recent research among physicians, nurses, nutritionists and pharmacists showed adequate knowledge (average 66% on the knowledge test), less confidence (55%) but noted a serious lack of communication skills (average 2.2 out of 10) regarding herbs and nutritional supplements. Athletic trainers and coaches were found to be reasonably knowledge-able, especially those working with female athletes and having more than 15 years of experience.

Supplement Types and Undesirable Consequences

A central issue in researching supplement use is the paucity of regulatory control of supplement providers coupled to a poor understanding within the user community. However, in broad terms many supplements have been associated, rightly or wrongly, with performance enhancement and health maintenance including: caffeine, ephedrine, creatine, whey protein, antioxidants, ginseng, multivitamins, vitamin C, iron, Echinacea and magnesium supplements.

Table: Supplements taken by high performance athletes.

Listed by product/brand names	Listed by components/contents
Ache Free, Cyclone, Build Up, Green Magic, Herbalife, Hydroxycut, Immune Support, Kalms, Lactibiane, Leppin, Lucozade, Met-Rx, Minadex, Mega EPA, MSN, Multibionta, Musashi Protein, Qlo, Slim Fast, SportsFlex, Vitabalance	Aloe Vera, Alpha-lipoic Acid, Amino Acids, Arnica, Black strap molas-ses, Calcium, Calendula, Carbohydrate & recovery drinks, C-Glutamine, Chinese Tea, Chromium, Chondroitin, CLA (conjugated linoleic acid), Cod liver oil, Coenzyme Q10, Colostrum, Cranberry juice tablets, Diges-tive enzymes, Dried skimmed milk powder, Echinacea tea bags, Elec-trolytes, Evening primrose oil, Ferrous gluconate, Fish oils, Flax seed oil, Folic acid, Garlic capsules, Glucosomine, Harpagophytum procum-bens, Hydroxybetamethylbutyrate, L-Carnitine, L-Glutamine, Maitake mushroom, Matltodextrin/Aspartame, meal replacement, Multi Min-eral Supplements, Olbas Oil, Protein drinks, Selenium, Soya protein, Starflower oil, Sumpast, Tribulous Terrestris, Vitamin B, B combined with Forceval capsules, Vitamin B complex, Vitamin D and E, Zinc

Beyond contaminated products that easily lead to adverse results in doping tests, vitamin products with accurately listed compounds and substances can also be harmful. High levels of vitamin and mineral intake can lead to toxic side effects. For example, the use of iron supplementation by elite athletes is not uncommon and whilst iron is beneficial for athletes with iron deficiency, it can also cause harm with long-term use or certain medical conditions. Similarly, excess intake of vitamin C can be harmful as well as in combination with iron, which may cause damage to the gastrointestinal tract (GI) and initiate or aggravate symptoms associated with chronic GI disorders. The long-term effects of creatine are still unknown but short term side-effects such as cramping and dehydration have been reported along with the suggestion for its use to be under medical supervision. Caffeine is no longer on the list of the IOC's prohibited substances. However, as athletes can use it in training and competition, the relationship between caffeine intake and resulting side-effects such as high blood pressure warrant further study. Whilst the controversial natural stimulant, ephedrine, has a threshold (concentration in the urine exceeds 10 µg/ml) for consideration for doping, the serious harm, which may be caused by ephedrine is well documented and the direct evidence eventually led to a ban on ephedrine in 2004 by Food and Drug Administration (FDA), USA. While the use of blood doping and erythropoietin (EPO) are prohibited, cobalt is not included in the World Anti Doping Association's list of prohibited substances. Cobalt produces similar effects to hypoxia and results in enhanced erythropoiesis, thus in improved sport performance but such practice may be harmful.

Existing data sets that include both 'supplements' and 'rationale/knowledge' variables can be used to obtain evidence regarding athletes' potentially dangerous, incongruent behaviour. Rationale or knowledge can also be replaced by behavioural intention or beliefs about particular substances. Practically, any data that allow a scientifically and statistically meaningful contingency table to be formed are suitable for such analyses. It is suggested that existing, recent, large-scale national surveys conducted among adult and adolescent athletes by national level sport organisations and governing bodies should be scrutinised to test the hypothesis regarding supplement use in sports.

By creating a series of two by two contingency tables from cross-tabling each supplement intake categories and reasons for supplement use, we can:

- Test for relationships between answers (i.e., testing for independence of the two variables).

- Estimate the strength of this relationship from the proportion of congruent pairs of answers (reasons given for supplement use matches with the reported supplement use).

- Calculate the relative proportion of answers indicating informed choices and incongruent answers (reasons given for supplement use are not followed by the appropriate supplement) and compare the observed pattern of supplement use to an expected pattern.

- Test whether this pattern characterises the athlete population.

A pair of answers is congruent if there is an agreement between an athlete's self-reported supplement use and rationale. The connection is not explicitly made by the athlete but calculated afterwards from answers given on two separate and seemingly independent questions. In surveys of supplement use, athletes are often asked about the substances they have had experience with and some of these surveys also contain explicit questions regarding the reasons behind supplement taking. For instance, a group of athletes were asked: i) whether they use supplements to increase their strength and power output; and ii) if they take creatine – a substance known for this effect and currently not sanctioned in competitive sport. Answer options to both questions were limited to dichotomous (Yes/No) responses, thus its contingency table is a two-by-two square. Assume that exactly 100 athletes were asked and 75% of them take supplements to maintain or increase strength. In an ideal case when all athletes make an informed and rational decision about supplements, we would expect X to be 75 and W to be 25, whereas both Y and Z should be zero. This {75, 0, 25, 0} is the expected pattern under the assumption of the fully informed choice. On the contrary, a pattern of $X = 0$, $Z = 75$, $Y = 25$ and $W = 0$ would indicate a great deal of confusion or complete misinformation about supplements and their physiological effects.

However, in real life it is not likely that we can observe a perfect pattern, thus we use appropriate statistical analyses to determine whether the observed pattern significantly differs from: i) what is expected; or ii) what would happen by random chance if we assume that the two questions are unrelated. Descriptive statistics obtained from the sample are very interesting and informative but no inferences can be made to the population from which the sample was drawn.

Adverse Effects of Sports Supplement on Men

The illicit use of prohibited drugs (i.e. doping) is unfortunately very often underestimated by both amateur and professional athletes, are known to disrupt at different levels and throughout various mechanisms the male hypothalamic-pituitary-gonadal axis, resulting in hypogonadism and infertility.

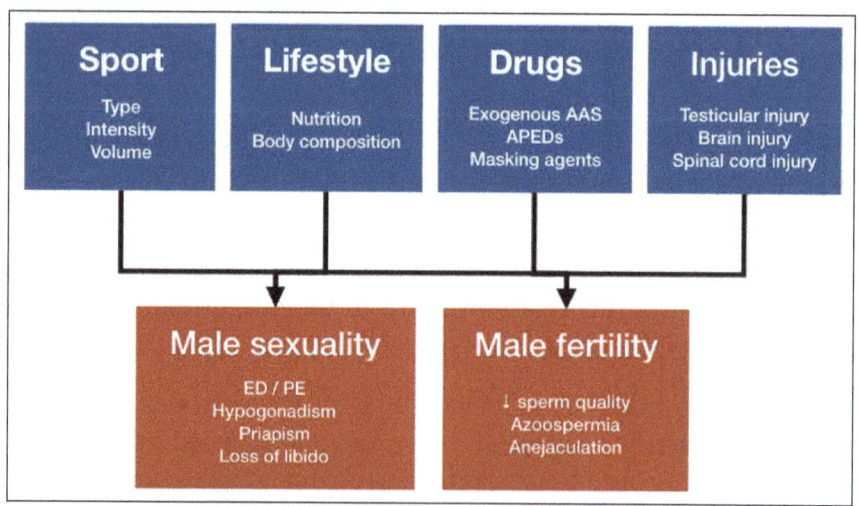

Disorders of male sexual and reproductive functions in athletes. Abbreviations: AAS, androgenic anabolic steroids; APEDs, appearance and performance-enhancing drugs; ED, erectile dysfunction; PE, premature ejaculation.

Lifestyle interventions have been proven to be effective as the first step towards a good general health and even for maintaining adequate reproductive and sexual health. Physical exercise is widely considered to be one of the bases of a healthy lifestyle. However, contrary to popular belief, "being fit" does not necessarily mean "being healthy". Solid evidence has suggested that adequate regular physical activity (i.e. physical exercise, sports, etc.) might have positive effects on cardio-vascular, endocrine, metabolic and neurological status, whereas different forms of excessive and strenuous physical training often have deleterious effects on both general and reproductive health. Furthermore, the widespread use of doping substances in general population and in both professional and non-professional athletes has become a worrying phenomenon in terms of health risk. Many people abuse hormones in order to provide better outcomes for their physical appearance, while – despite increasing efforts from the World Anti-Doping Agency (WADA) athletes are constantly looking for new drugs to improve their sports performance.

Physical exercise and sports have been observed to have the potential for affecting human's reproduction (i.e., reproduction-related sexual behavior and fertility), in both positive and negative ways. In males, sexual and spermatogenetic functions might be maintained or improved by adequate physical activity, whereas impairments in sexuality and in fertility have been observed following excessive training and drug abuse (i.e. doping).

Physical Exercise, Sports and the Male Hypothalamic-pituitary-gonadal Axis

The physiology of male reproduction is the result of fine tuning between several hormones involved in sexual function and spermatogenesis. For such purpose, the hypothalamus, pituitary and testes act together; therefore, it's common practice to describe them as a single entity, namely the hypothalamic-pituitary-gonadal (HPG) axis. After puberty, pulsatile release of gonadotropin-releasing hormone (GnRH) from hypothalamic GnRH-secreting neurons stimulates production of luteinizing hormone (LH) and follicle-stimulating hormone (FSH) from secretory cells of the anterior pituitary; in males, FSH and LH act on the testes, stimulating spermatogenesis and testosterone production respectively. Secretion of GnRH is regulated by negative feedback mechanisms involving inhibin B, and both direct and indirect action from testosterone. Energy balance dynamically regulates endogenous HPG axis, which in turn also regulates both exercise performance and success in competition; unsurprisingly, both reduced androgen secretion and excessive levels of testosterone might have deleterious effects on performance as well as on general health.

Physical Exercise, Sports and Testosterone: The Good

Testosterone is a widely-known determinant of muscle volume, strength, function and adaptation to exercise-related stress in humans (e.g. athletes, amateurs, and so forth), whether young or older; however, its role goes further beyond, as testosterone might influence body composition, cognitive processes, glucose and protein metabolism, erythropoiesis and reproductive function in both athletes and non-athletes. Its effects are patent when employing it in replacement therapy in hypogonadal subjects.

Table: Physiological effects of testosterone on adaptation to physical exercise and sports performance in males.

Somatic Growth	Control of growth
	Epiphyseal cartilage closure
	Secondary sexual characteristics
	Somatic masculinization

Endocrine-metabolic system	Anti-cortisol effects (metabolism, steroid receptor competition)
	Increased anaerobic glycolytic capacity
	Increased enzymes activity in mitochondria
	Increased phosphocreatine content
	Increased protein anabolism
	Increased sarco-tubular enzymes activity
	Inhibited stress related CRH-ACTH-Cortisol response
	Pro-insulin and insulin-like effects
	Reduced protein catabolism
	Stimulated erythropoiesis
	Synergic effects with growth hormone
Functional capacity	Increased aerobic and anaerobic capacity
	Cardiovascular efficiency
	Increased muscle strength and explosive strength
	Increased muscle adaptation to training
Body composition	Increased bone mineral density
	Increased muscle mass
	Male pattern muscle distribution
	Reduced fat mass
Central nervous system	Increased aggressiveness
	Increased dominance
	Increased inclination to command
	Increased motivation to compete
	Increased neuro-muscular conduction
	Increased visual-spatial capacities
	Reduced empathy
	Reduced negative reaction to external rapid stimuli and alarms
	Reduced perception of negative emotions
	Reduced sense of fatigue
Psycho-motor and sports capacity	Increased aggressiveness in competition
	Increased motivation to compete
	Increased resistance to fatigue
	Increased visual-spatial orientation during competition

Despite lacking evidence in regards to exact mechanisms involved, acute maximal and sub-maximal physical exercise may lead to a rapid increase in serum testosterone concentration, likely resulting in better adaptation and performance in both muscle activity and functional capacity during physical exercise. Physical exercise and sports competition act as a stressor, and testosterone is likely acting as a homeostatic agent, together with the whole range of hormones secreted during or shortly after physical exercise. Enhanced pituitary responsiveness, improved Leydig function, reduced testosterone clearance and changes in testicular blood flow have all been investigated as possible causes; however, no definite evidence has been obtained so far, suggesting that a combination of mechanisms is the most likely explanation. The endocrine response to exercise related stress is related to various factors (e.g. type, intensity and duration of physical activity, etc.)

Physical Exercise, Sports and Testosterone: The Bad

The acute exercise often leads to a transient increase in testosterone levels; on the contrary, a marked decrease in testosterone levels has been suggested in athletes undergoing chronic exercise. Incorrectly executed exercise or poorly developed training programs elicit negative endocrine responses and physiological consequences. The chronic exposure to excessive loads of endurance training may impair the function of the HPG axis, leading to significantly and persistently reduced basal (resting-state) free and total testosterone levels, often remaining within the physiological range, with no concurrent increase in LH levels. The resulting clinical and biochemical phenotype depicts the "exercise-hypogonadal male condition", as defined by Hackney and colleagues; the pathophysiology of this condition have not been fully elucidated, although pituitary GnRH resistance, increased prolactin secretion and inhibitory effects on LH secretion from ghrein and leptin have all been considered as possible "triggers". Retrospective studies have often shown a reduction of free and total testosterone concentrations in endurance-trained men, whereas prospective studies have often failed to provide definite results because of the varying features of the training period, the magnitude of training stimulus and the volume of training load employed.

To the present date, several authors have reported the effects of short-term and long-term intensive training: significantly decreased concentrations of total and free testosterone, as well as reduced FSH and LH secretion/pulsatility, and increased SHBG levels have been reported following high-intensity exercise. More recently, cortisol and testosterone dynamics following exhaustive endurance exercise have been described in endurance-trained males, suggesting that recovery from endurance exercise sessions at ventilatory threshold might require up to 72 h for free testosterone to return to baseline values. Previous findings in high-altitude marathon runners and professional cyclists provide further confirmation with regards to the effects of different kinds of exercise on testosterone secretion and profile.

Whether testosterone suppression is the result of a physiological adaptation to stress or an undesirable side effect of excessive training is a matter still open to debate. The best treatment for exercise-induced hypogonadism is to reduce exercise load; however, constant monitoring of androgen status is suggested in all athletes undergoing strenuous training in order to promptly address any issues related to testosterone deficiency.

Physical Exercise, Sports and Testosterone: The Ugly

Hormones, including testosterone, act on muscle strength, adaptation to exercise and recovery: therefore, untreated male athletes with testosterone deficiency are likely to incur in specific risks for health and for their physiological adaptation and performance during exercise. Male athletes affected by untreated hypogonadism with hypo-testosteronemia (e.g. congenital hypogonadotropic hypogonadism, Klinefelter Syndrome, anorchia, and so forth) in association to worse results in terms of performance and adaptation to physical exercise and sports are more likely affected by increased risks for general health, ranging from osteoporotic fractures to cardiovascular accidents related to the combination of hypo-testosteronemia with high exercise-strain. Testosterone deficiency is also, of course, an issue for all ages: hypogonadism is rarely overtly symptomatic in athletes but may become a primary cause for concern in older subjects.

Given its properties, testosterone is in the WADA list of prohibited substances, and therefore athletes in need of treatment should obtain a Therapeutic Use Exemption (TUE) according to the WADA criteria by the respective NADO. To prevent misuse, both clinicians and athletes should respect the official therapeutic indications and authorized formulations/doses. This procedure does not differ from others needed for other pathologies such as diabetes mellitus and adrenal insufficiency.

Sports, Sexual Function and Fertility in Male Athletes

Sexual Function

Reduced global physical exercise (i.e. sedentary behavior) is considered a risk factor for several chronic diseases and conditions, including sexual dysfunction in males; therefore, it should come as no surprise that adequate physical activity is fundamental to maintain or improve sexual health and that physical activity and the level of physical fitness are both associated to the quality of erectile function. Better sexual health is closely associated with improvements in sexual activity and reproductive capacity. Lifestyle modifications, including physical exercise, are in fact suggested as a first-line treatment for erectile dysfunction, since exercise improves bioavailability of nitric oxide and increases the number of endothelial progenitor cells, while at the same time diminishing concentrations of markers of oxidative stress and expression of TNF-α, IL-1-beta and IL-6, therefore improving endothelial function and consequently reducing the risk for erectile dysfunction. Two recent meta-analysis studies have proven the benefits of moderate, or moderate-to-vigorous healthy physical activity on erectile function, in both short-term and long-term interventions as well as in trials evaluating physical activity and exercise alone or in addition to usual care; however, suggesting that all kinds of physical exercise improve sexual health is misleading, as clearly proven in female athletes suffering from the "female athlete triad" – a syndrome featuring low energy availability, menstrual dysfunction, and low bone mineral density, frequently observed in a variety of sports. Some analogies between female and male athletes have been described in regards to bone health and nutritional deficiencies, but there are also similarities concerning sexual dysfunctions in both sexes. Male athletes suffering from exercise-induced hypogonadism are more likely to develop erectile dysfunction and ejaculatory disorders, as both conditions are also closely associated with reduced testosterone. Reduced sexual drive is among the classical symptoms of androgen deficiency, and testosterone supplementation is likely to improve sexual function in hypogonadal subjects; however, a reduced exercise load is the suggested treatment in athletes suffering from exercise-induced hypogonadism, although unrealistic for athletes whose ultimate goal is to compete and win.

Premature ejaculation (PE) is the most common male sexual dysfunction, with an estimated prevalence ranging from 8 to 30% up to 22–38% in all age groups. The pathogenesis of PE is complex, possibly involving psychological disturbances, alterations in hormonal status and lower urinary tract infections; however, in regards to erectile disorders, lifestyles seem to heavily influence orgasmic function. A negative association has been recently described between physical activity and PE, suggesting that PE is more likely to occur in patients reporting lower levels of physical exercise: this preliminary finding, however, deserves attention since the significance of the association did not change despite correction for age, erectile dysfunction, alcohol use and body mass index.

Fertility

Physically active subjects are more likely to have better sexual health, and are therefore more likely to have sexual activity; however, despite the "need" to have sex in order to conceive, the issue of male fertility is a separate entity, requiring a completely different approach. Male fertility is remarkably affected by a variety of lifestyle factors, exerting either positive or negative effects on spermatogenesis. Smoking, alcohol use, sedentary behavior are known risk factors for male infertility; however, how physical exercise may relate to male infertility is still unclear as contradictory results in different studies have been found to date.

Different kinds of physical activity characterized by a different exercise load, might have different effects on sperm parameters. The positive effects of an active lifestyle on spermatogenesis have been confirmed by comparing sperm parameters of physically active and sedentary men; higher levels (in the normal range) of FSH, LH and testosterone have been described in physically active subjects compared to sedentary subjects. More recent reports have concluded that moderate training is associated with improvements in sperm DNA integrity and semen quality and with reduced expression of seminal markers of inflammation and oxidative stress. However, once again, deleterious consequences for spermatogenesis have been repeatedly described following intensive exercise loads; worse morphology and concentration have been described in triathletes compared to physically active subjects and water polo players, therefore suggesting that more strenuous feats might actually prove harmful to spermatogenesis and sperm DNA integrity, and even seminal antioxidant capacity. In some of the early years De Souza and colleagues already hypothesized a volume threshold to start observing reproductive alterations, besides the other findings already described both an increase in reactive oxygen species (ROS) production and a decrease in ROS scavengers have been described after 16 weeks of intensive cycling training in humans as well as in animal models reflecting apoptotic events on the spermatogenic lineage. Cycling more than 5 h per week has been associated with a decline in both sperm concentration and motility.

Evidence would once again seem to suggest that moderate, healthy exercise is the key for a better overall health, whereas excessive loads of endurance training are more likely to induce worse outcomes, also in terms of fertility.

Besides volume and intensity, several factors might affect male fertility in athletes. Physical exercise is often suggested as a means for weight loss: in regards to male fertility, this has proven useful in improving sperm parameters. However, adequate physical activity is only moderately useful for assisted reproduction techniques, as improvements in sperm parameters do not always mirror clinical outcomes (i.e. clinical pregnancy or live birth rates). Furthermore, excessive training might result in worse sperm parameters, possibly negatively affecting the chances of successful treatment. It should be taken into account that professional athletes perform higher absolute volumes of training at top-end intensity compared with amateur athletes; nevertheless, the same relative intensity elicits less physical stress on professional athletes compared to amateur ones. Training intensity should be considered different according to the athlete's status. Furthermore, professional athletes may be more prone to evaluate training intensity according to parameters different from heart rate, which is affected by many variables (i.e stimulants, diet, hydration status, sports, temperature).

Table: Levels of risk based on physical activity volume and intensity.

Volume (hours/week) and intensity	Level of Risk
+30 h training or racing/weeks including moderate and high intensity	Very high risk
20–30 h training or racing/weeks including moderate and high intensity	High risk
10–20 h training or racing/weeks including moderate and high intensity	Medium risk
5–15 h training or racing/weeks not including moderate and high intensity	Low risk
Less than 5 h training or racing/weeks not including moderate and high intensity	Very low risk

Table: Training Intensity for amateur athletes.

Intensity	% Heart rate Reserve (HRR) or % oxygen uptake reserve (VO$_2$R)	% Heart rate (HR) max	% maximum oxygen uptake (VO$_2$max)
Very low	< 30	< 57	< 37
Low	30–39	57–63	37–45
Moderate	40–59	64–76	46–63
High	60–89	77–95	64–90
Very High (Elite training)	> 90	> 96	> 91

Table: Training intensity for elite athletes.

Intensity	% Heart rate (HR) max	% maximum oxygen uptake (VO$_2$ max)	Ventilatory Threshold (VT)	Blood Lactate Levels (mM)	Lactate Threshold (LT)
Very low	54–73	50–65	< VT 1	< 1.2	< LT 1
Low	74–83	66–80		1.3–2.0	
Moderate	84–88	81–87	VT 1 – VT 2	2.1–3.6	LT 1 – LT 2
High	89–93	88–93		4.3–5.7	
Very High (Elite training)	> 94	94–100	> VT 2	> 5.8	> LT 2

Potential Mechanisms Involved in Negative Effects of Physical Activity on Male Fertility

Despite a solid body of evidence proving that excessive physical exercise might negatively affect male fertility, there is little knowledge concerning the potential mechanisms involved in the decrease of sperm quality. Exercise-induced hypogonadism is likely to occur in a minority of athletes; therefore, several hypotheses have been postulated in order to correctly address this issue. Any increase in scrotal temperature is likely to impair spermatogenesis by induction of germ cell death: mechanisms include autophagy, DNA damage and apoptosis. Everyday clothing is supposed to have an effect on spermatogenesis: tight undertrousers provide significantly more heat to testes compared to loose-fitting ones, a phenomenon seemingly attenuated by walking because of perigenital air circulation. Whether more intense physical activity is associated with increased scrotal temperature is still a matter for debate. Exercise-induced hypoxia has been described in exercise training, as well as in aging; testicular dysfunction observed in high-altitude exercise is possibly associated with reduced oxygen availability, and might impair male fertility resulting in reduced sperm concentration. Similar reports have also addressed the effects of deep saturation dive on male fertility: negative effects on sperm motility and concentration were observed shortly after the dive and remained consistent up to 3 months later, suggesting that hyperbaric conditions are likely to impair spermatogenesis. Pudendal nerve compression, repeated trauma on the pelvic floor and other morpho-functional alterations commonly observed in cycling have been considered possible causes of male infertility as well.

Morpho-functional Alterations and Reproduction in Male Athletes

Some kinds of sports have been closely associated with male HPG morpho-functional alterations ultimately resulting in worse sexual function and reduced fertility. Brain and spinal cord injuries, as well as local trauma, are often cited as the most prevalent sports-related morpho-functional alterations possibly leading to erectile dysfunction and male infertility.

Traumatic brain injuries, as observed in football players and in kickboxers, may lead to long-term impairment of pituitary secretion, most often acutely presenting as isolated GH deficiency but possibly involving multiple axes during follow-up. Causes of hypopituitarism following concussion are still unknown: there are a few hypotheses in these regards, suggesting a role of hemorrhage, edema, autoimmunity or inflammatory and hypoxic state.

Pudendal nerve compression due to cycling is another complex, interesting phenomenon often resulting in urogenital complications. Either because of mechanical pressure, transient hypoxemia, or arterial insufficiency, ischemic neuropathy is likely to occur in cyclists; this might provide an explanation to the increased odds ratio for erectile dysfunction in people cycling more than 3 h per week. Cycling has also been associated with chronic prostatitis, a condition affecting both sexual and reproductive health. High-flow priapism is similarly more prevalent in cyclists: exercise-induced vascular trauma resulting in arterial-venous shunt is the most common etiology for this condition.

Increased abdominal pressure supposedly aggravates the development of varicocele in males. Rigano et al. reported significantly increased prevalence of higher grades of varicocele among athletes compared to non-athletes, with more severe forms affecting those training more than 6 h per week. Physical activity might also be an aggravating factor for athletes with varicocele: despite there being no statistically significant difference in sperm parameters between healthy athletes and controls, varicocele seems to be associated with worse outcomes in athletes compared to non-athletes in terms of sperm morphology. All athletes with varicocele should be clinically monitored, and treatment should be proposed if needed in order to preserve fertility and guarantee safe sport participation. More recently, Zampieri and Dall'Agnola suggested that sports practice might facilitate progression to clinical varicocele only in subjects affected by subclinical forms of varicocele.

Sports-related spinal cord injuries (SCIs) are uncommon outcomes of physical activity, although their rate is remarkably higher in some kinds of sports, such as rugby, diving and horseback riding. The incidence of SCIs has dramatically reduced in the last decades; however, the devastating effect on the involved athletes' quality of life has often rekindled media attention in these regards. Spinal trauma may result in different clinical syndromes based on the location of the lesion and on subsequent secondary events, such as hemorrhage and edema. SCIs most frequently occur in young, male athletes as compared to female athletes and impair the ability to obtain erection and to achieve ejaculation. Parasympathetic fibers originating from S2-S4 and entering the corpora cavernosa are needed for erectile function; patients with SCIs often lose psychogenic erections but may maintain reflexogenic erections, although this rarely allows for intercourse. Both sympathetic fibers from segments T10-L2 and somatic fibers from segments S2-S4 are involved in the ejaculatory reflex; more in detail, fibers from the segments T11-L2 transmit a signal via the hypogastric nerve plexus ultimately resulting in emission. Semen samples might still be collected, either through penile vibratory stimulation or via electro-ejaculation, and might often represent the only chance for fatherhood for these subjects.

Last, but not least, the issue of pelvic trauma deserves attention: in fact, more than half of testicular injuries occur during physical activity, most often as a result of blunt force trauma. In the most severe circumstances the resulting testicular damage might lead to primary hypogonadism; furthermore, the creation of anti-sperm autoantibodies might also affect male fertility. Testicular torsion usually presents without any previous traumatic injuries to the scrotum, with only 4–8% of cases resulting from trauma; however, some kinds of physical activity, most notably cycling, are linked to an increased risk of testicular torsion. Potential mechanisms resulting in testicular torsion are the repeated up-and-down movements of the legs, contraction of the cremasteric muscles and exaggerated cremasteric reflex. Blunt force trauma applied to the perineum might also result in penile injuries, although much less commonly than testicular injuries.

Doping, Sexual Function and Fertility in Male Athletes

The "doping epidemics" has crossed the boundaries of elite sports, and now appeals to a wide audience of subjects – from medal-winning athletes aiming to excel in competitions, to amateurs aiming to improve their looks without effort, "appearance and performance-enhancing drugs" (APEDs) use is widespread and seemingly increasing in recent years. The WADA has been actively involved in doping control, and several athletes have been sanctioned for doping use; however, the issue with APEDs lies not only in the effects on performance, but also in the possible – and often misjudged – side effects associated with their use. Furthermore, many supplements have hormone-related effects despite being advertised as "natural compounds", or might affect the endocrine milieu through indirect pathways, possibly by tampering with the "biological clock" and therefore acting as endocrine disruptors.

Table: Doping agents and their effects on male sexual and reproductive health.

Substance(s)	Used	Effects			
		Sexual desire	Erectile function	Ejaculatory function	Male fertility
Androgenic anabolic steroids	– for ergogenic and anabolic actions – for effects on CNS (↑aggressiveness, ↑ competitiveness...)	↑ or ↓	↓	↓ (delayed ejaculation, anejaculation)	↓
β-blockers	– to ↓ anxiety – to ↓ tremors – to ↓ heart rate		↓	↓ (delayed ejaculation, anejaculation)	
Diuretics	as masking agents for bodybuilding		↓	↓ (delayed ejaculation, anejaculation)	
Amphetamine, stimulants	for effects on CNS (↑aggressiveness, ↑ competitiveness) for (unproven) ergogenic properties	↑ or ↓	↓	↑ or ↓ (premature delayed or ejaculation, anejaculation)	↓

Testosterone and Androgenic Anabolic Steroids

It is widely accepted that administration of exogenous testosterone and of other androgenic anabolic steroids (AAS) exerts a suppressive effect on the HPG axis. Sexual and reproductive health are often impaired as a result of AAS-induced hypogonadism. Erectile dysfunction might be the first symptom of prolonged AAS abuse for subjects who are not interested in their fertility: clinicians should therefore pay attention to signs of AAS-induced hypogonadism during clinical assessment. Erectile dysfunction often occurs during the "post-cycle" period in abusers, when serum testosterone reaches its minimum, and is often associated with use of some AAS, most notably nandrolone.

Up to 2% of cases of male infertility can be explained by AAS abuse, whereas the vast majority of behavior-related infertility in female athletes is the result of excessive exercise. Unsurprisingly, low levels of FSH are closely associated with reduced sperm count; clinically, prolonged abuse of AAS is likely to induce testicular shrinkage because of tubular atrophy, due to HPG axis suppression. Studies in animal models have also suggested possible effects of AAS on male germ line apoptosis, as observed via TUNEL, caspase-3 assay and transmission electron microscopy. Compared to erectile function, reproductive function is less likely to be permanently impaired by AAS: for most people spontaneous resolution of AAS-induced oligozoospermia and azoospermia has been observed in less than a year after discontinuation of APEDs.

AAS suppress intra-testicular testosterone production by inhibition of the HPG axis: therefore, selective estrogen receptor modulators (SERMs) and gonadotropins have been used in order to quicken recovery following AAS cessation, but individual response to treatment is highly variable and therefore difficult to assess. Several factors complicate the assessment of the effects of AAS on reproductive and sexual function, such as multi-drug regimens "stacking" several molecules and depot effects: for the same reasons, recovery may take a long time, even 12–24 months following prompt discontinuation of APEDs. More severe effects might occur in patients abusing AAS in puberty, as changes in the HPG axis in this time frame might lead to long-lasting damage on sexual health and development. In these regards, several treatments have been proposed for AAS-induced hypogonadism: SERMs such as clomiphene citrate 25 mg on alternate days have been successfully used for management of low testosterone, possibly after a 4-week tapered course of testosterone replacement therapy for more severe cases. Should testosterone levels fail to rise despite treatment, primary testicular failure should be suspected and recovery is limited. Recent reports on hCG-based combined treatment seem to suggest that the vast majority of cases of testosterone-related azoospermia or oligozoospermia would benefit from treatment, with no significant difference in regards to supplemental therapies. Another issue lies in the frequent use of multi-drug regimens: athletes often "mix" AAS and other substances, most notably hCG, in order to reduce the suppression on the HPG axis or in hopes of synergies between treatments. Little evidence has been published in these regards, but reports suggest that conjoined administration of hCG and AAS impairs fertility, similarly to what has been described in AAS-only abusers. In addition, we highlight that it is not known if and how the large use and abuse of not prohibited substances (e.g. supplements, ergogenic aids and drugs) in athletes (i.e. not considered doping), often associated to the assumption of prohibited substances (i.e. doping), could influence the reproductive axis.

A question largely left unanswered is whether administration of AAS during puberty is likely to impair spermatogenesis: reports from over-tall boys treated with high doses of testosterone seem to suggest that recovery time is not different from non-treated subjects, but evidence is inconsistent and caution is therefore advised.

Non-hormonal Drugs used for Performance and Appearance Enhancement

Despite being significantly less common than AAS, several substances have been used in different sports in order to enhance performance; however, negative effects of these drugs have been reported concerning sexual and reproductive function. Beta-blockers, often used in order to reduce anxiety and tremors in precision sports, are likely to worsen erectile function; furthermore, in vitro studies have reported inhibitory effects of beta-blockers on smooth muscle in reproductive tracts, possibly resulting in delayed ejaculation or, in the most severe cases, anejaculation. In regards to cardiovascular treatments, diuretics, most notably thiazides, might impair erectile function: these drugs are sometimes used by athletes in order as masking agents for concomitant treatments, but use of these drugs by bodybuilders aiming to improve their physical appearance is an increasingly worrying phenomenon and their possible side effects might be amplified by coexisting eating disorders. Amphetamines and stimulants – including some over the counter treatments, such as pseudoephedrine – are used for their effects on the central nervous system: by enhancing reflexes, increasing aggressiveness and (possibly) having ergogenic effects, these drugs are ideal candidates as doping agents in sports involving short bursts of speed or strength. Among their side effects, these substances might both enhance or worsen erectile function, sexual drive and ejaculatory latency; in animal models, testicular damage resulting in impaired fertility has been described in rats treated with amphetamine, suggesting a negative effect on spermatogenesis as well. Carnitine, a compound with reported antioxidant properties, is often used as an APED; while some effects on sperm parameters have been reported in several in vivo studies using less than 3 g/day, there is no evidence on the effects of high carnitine intake on male fertility. Similarly, several other compounds are often used for performance enhancing purposes, such as amino acids and soy or milk proteins. Some authors have reported negative effects of soy proteins on male fertility, although other studies have suggested otherwise; likewise, creatine and other compounds commonly used by athletes, have not been adequately investigated in regards to their possible effects on spermatogenesis and fertility.

Nutritional Supplements and Doping

The current preoccupation with nutritional supplements demonstrated by many athletes is a reflection of certain societal trends, the presence and persistence of an aggressive, unregulated supplement industry, and the failure of many sport organizations, sport scientists, and physicians to provide appropriate education regarding the nutritional basis of athletic activity. Supplement use in the absence of a specific need, deficiency, or disease is not recommended. While increased ingestion of creatine has been shown to produce small changes in performance in very specific exercise conditions, the expectations of athletes for performance enhancement have been described as "inordinate." Increased intake of carbohydrates prior to (carbohydrate loading), during, and after exercise has been noted to improve and sustain performance; the ingestion of caffeine has also been shown to delay fatigue and improve physical performance.

The use of dietary supplements has been increasing significantly in the population at large, and it is perhaps not surprising that athletes should reflect this trend. But it is ironic that for many in sport, nutrition seems now to be a religion rather than a science; it has been the experience of both authors that many athletes, their coaches, and other advisors hold views regarding nutrition that are not scientific, sound, or sensible. No benefits have been demonstrated for many of the products avidly consumed by some athletes. Yet it is clear that an enormous appetite for such products has been created. Some athletes at the Sydney 2000 Olympic games were consuming as many as 18–20 different supplements daily; one competitor ingested 25 separate items each day.

The introduction in 1994 of the "Dietary Supplement and Health Education Act" (DSHEA) in the U.S. has unleashed an industry, a multitude of hucksters, and selfstyled nutritional "advisors" whose products are widely advertised, particularly on the Internet, in ways that are often both grandiose and misleading. As a consequence of this legislation, it is now virtually impossible to ascertain the accuracy and validity of the labeling, content, source, or manufacturer of many commonly advertised products. It is important to understand that there is no longer, as a consequence of the passage of the DSHEA, any independent, government regulation of these products. That such products are often advertised beneath a veneer of pseudoscientific information mixed with a variety of glowing "endorsations" serves to confuse athletes even more.

It is known that many nutritional supplements are inadvertently or deliberately contaminated with substances that may cause athletes to test positive when subjected to doping controls. In such instances, it is typical that the products in question contain stimulants, steroids, or steroidal precursors. Millions of men and women are noted to be "currently using potent drugs, widely sold over the counter as 'supplements,' despite their known adverse effects, unknown long-term risks, and possible potential for causing abuse or dependence." Sport physicians and scientists, as well as sport administrators, must understand the complexities of the current situation and develop strategies and approaches that will permit athletes and others to appreciate both the lack of any necessity for the use of many supplements and the hazards that may be associated with their use. Principal among such strategies is the recognition that only appropriately qualified professionals should be providing nutritional assessments and guidance to athletes. The sport community is awash with a variety of individuals whose credibility and credentials in the area of sport and nutrition are suspect or self-ordained.

Supplements and Anabolic Steroids

The detection of the use of anabolic steroids is based on the presence of the banned steroid, its metabolites, or a distortion of the ratio of testosterone to epitestosterone (the T/E ratio) in a urine sample. It is critical to this discussion to understand that certain steroid products available as "supplements" in the U.S. are metabolized to compounds that also are produced by the metabolism of banned anabolic steroids—19-norandrosterone, produced both by the metabolism of 19-nortestosterone (Nandrolone) or 19-norandrostenedione, is the best example of such a metabolite. Currently, the presence above a certain level (2 ng/ml in males, 5 ng/ml in females) of 19-norandrosterone in a urine sample will result in a positive doping test as it is deemed to be indicative of the use of 19-nortestosterone (Nandrolone), a banned anabolic steroid. In the past 10 years, the percentage of samples reported positive by International Olympic Committee (IOC)-accredited laboratories for 19-norsteroids accounted for approximately 0.25% of all specimens tested.12

Clearly it is important that athletes understand the implications of consuming "supplements" that contain steroid precursors. Sadly, it cannot be assumed that only steroid "supplements" or products containing or presumed to contain precursor compounds place an athlete at risk for testing positive. An array of other "nonhormonal" supplements also have been noted to contain steroids or precursor products (creatine, tribulus terrestris, carnitine, chrysin, various "vitamins," minerals, and herbal extracts) distributed in numerous countries have been found to be contaminated with 19- norsteroids in amounts sufficient to cause a positive doping test. The risks of consuming such products only can be reduced when the manufacture of nutritional supplements is appropriately and rigorously regulated.

It has been possible for a number of years for athletes to purchase a variety of androgens, prohormones, or precursors such as DHEA (dehydroepiandrosterone), androstenedione, androstenediol, 19-norandrostenedione, and 19-norandrostenediol either singly or in countless combinations. When marketed as dietary supplements, such products escape any form of regulation. It is revealing to note that an analysis of 16 different preparations of DHEA found that the content of this steroid varied from 0% to 150% of the dosage indicated on the product label; three of the products contained no DHEA whatsoever. More troubling for sport physicians and sport organizations is the fact that products containing androstenedione have been contaminated with amounts of 19-norandrostenedione sufficient to cause positive doping tests. The issue of steroid precursors came to the forefront in North America in 1998 when the use of androstenedione by a professional baseball player, Mark McGwire, became the subject of media scrutiny and public criticism. Marketed as a so-called "dietary supplement," this steroidal precursor is widely available from a variety of sources in North America and elsewhere. It is alleged that sales of this product increased dramatically following the revelation of its use by this well-known professional athlete. It is also quite clearly forbidden by the IOC and all International Sport Federations, and in the U.S.A. by the National Football League and the National Collegiate Athletic Association.

Norandrostenedione, norandrostenediol, and nortestosterone (Nandrolone) are metabolized and excreted as norandrosterone and noretiocholanolone, as has been discussed. Urine samples collected after the use of such substances will test positive as noted above and, characteristically, an athlete will immediately express surprise and innocence at the revelation of a positive test. A careful investigation of more than 150 nonhormonal sport supplements provided by athletes (who blamed their use for failing a doping test) revealed that steroids not listed on the label contaminated 18 preparations produced by 12 different manufacturers. Testosterone, itself a strictly regulated substance and therefore not freely available, has been identified as a contaminant and, in fact, the principal constituent of some hormonal "supplements." Even those "supplement" products that clearly indicate that they contain a steroid are found to fail even the minimal standards of the DSHEA: 11 of 12 brands, containing 8 different steroids, were found to contain less than the amounts listed on the label; one brand contained testosterone.

It is clear that those athletes who consume products that contain steroid and steroid precursor products, notwithstanding that they are marketed as "nutritional supplements," place themselves at risk of testing positive in doping controls. This reality must be communicated to athletes and to those in their entourage. Experience suggests that this can be a very difficult task. Incredulous athletes are loath to consider that their "supplements" may produce a positive doping test, let alone that they are, in all likelihood, of insignificant or no nutritional value.

Supplements and Stimulants

In 1960, the amphetamine-related death of a Danish cyclist Knut Jensen catalyzed the development of antidoping programs and drug testing in sport. Since, and before, that time, the use of a variety of stimulants has been depressingly common in sport. Ironically, with perhaps two notable exceptions, caffeine and ephedrine, there is little evidence to support the contention that many common stimulants are capable of enhancing performance. Nevertheless athletes continue to ingest such compounds risking their health and positive doping tests in the process.

Caffeine

Caffeine is a ubiquitous substance, consumed daily by an overwhelming majority of the population in a variety of forms. Present in beverages, confectionery, pain medications, and in large numbers of dietary supplements, its use in sport is controlled by examining urine for its presence beyond a certain threshold level (12 ug/ml). There is strong evidence to support its ability to enhance performance at doses similar to those used in everyday life (which are highly unlikely to produce urine levels greater than the threshold). It has been conclusively demonstrated that doses of at least 9 mg/kg are required to result in the maximal allowable limit established by the IOC; doses as low as 2–3 mg/kg are effective in improving performance. There is marked interindividual variation in urinary caffeine concentrations following ingestion of the same caffeine dose, a fact that has important implications for an athlete and for those charged with developing the rules and regulations regarding doping control. There are suggestions that caffeine is actually ergolytic at high doses, presumably because of the production of agitation, tremors, and mental distraction. Because of its ability to impart a sense of energy and arousal, and its known capacity to accentuate endurance performance, caffeine is a favorite ingredient of dietary supplements. Such supplements are often marketed as aids to weight loss, fatigue prevention, and energy production. The presence of caffeine may not be noted on product labels or its presence may be "disguised" by the use of another identifier such as guarana or kola nut (which contain caffeine and other xanthines).

Athletes must use extreme caution when purchasing and using such products. The interindividual variations in caffeine metabolism, the unknown or concentrated quantities of caffeine in a supplement, and the ingestion of other forms of caffeine may produce elevated levels of urinary caffeine capable of producing a positive test result. This may be especially critical for younger athletes or those of small stature. It is possible that increased levels of caffeine may actually retard or impair performance. The inadequacies of the current regulation of nutritional supplements preclude the possibility of an athlete knowing, with confidence, the nature and quantity of the contents of any supplement product—hence the importance of ensuring, to the extent possible, that they understand the implications, and consider the necessity, of any supplement ingestion.

Ephedrine

Sympathomimetics such as ephedrine and related compounds have long been banned in sport. Structurally related to amphetamine, there is little evidence to support the contention that, with the exception of ephedrine, these products are capable of enhancing performance. Initial evaluations of the ergogenic properties of ephedrine did not demonstrate any ergogenic effects. More recently it has been shown that, particularly in association with caffeine, ephedrine can increase the duration of endurance exercise and enhance anaerobic performance. Ephedrine is prohibited in sport, and a positive doping test results if it is found in the urine at levels greater than 10 ug/ml.

Ephedrine is a very common constituent of nutritional supplements, and in particular is found in many products that are aggressively marketed to athletes. It is present in a broad array of products promoted to assist with weight loss or to increase athletic performance. Ephedrine is derived from ephedra-containing plant sources, and thus is often touted as a "natural" product. It is frequently identified as Ma Huang (Chinese ephedra), and in this guise (or others) may go unnoticed by consumers who may be wary of consuming ephedrine by virtue of cardiovascular or other concerns. Consumers have good reason to be cautious about the ingestion of ephedrine. Concerns about the safety of this compound continue to grow and reflect increasing evidence of the morbidity and mortality associated with its use. Cardiovascular problems predominate, particularly arrhythmias, myocardial infarctions, sudden death, seizures, and stroke. The deaths of young athletic individuals following the use of ephedrine-containing "performance-enhancing supplements," such as "Ripped Fuel" and "Ultimate Orange," is both tragic and ironic. It is unsettling to note that such problems can emerge in the absence of any preexisting cardiovascular disease, and do not appear to be dose related. Of equal concern is the realization that many individuals may develop an ephedrine dependency. Ephedrine-containing products also are suggested as being safe alternatives ("herbal ecstasy") to drugs like methylenedioxymethamphetamine (MDMA), and may be used by athletes unwilling to participate in the use of street drugs; neuropsychiatric and cardiovascular problems may follow. These tragedies, and the added concern that they may be under-reported, have caused both the DSHEA and the availability of ephedrine-containing products to come under attack. As is the case with all dietary supplements, variation may exist between the labeling and the actual contents of the product; some products fail to list the presence of ephedrine completely.

Athletes must exercise vigilance before purchasing, accepting, or ingesting any dietary supplement; not only may the unwitting (or calculated) consumption of ephedrine cause an athlete to test positive, there are also significant health consequences that may follow the use of such supplements.

The widespread availability and use of a multiplicity of so called "nutritional supplements" pose specific problems for athletes, coaches, and sport organizations alike. The appetite for such products, and the zealotry of those involved in encouraging their use, speaks poorly of the status of science in the preparation, training, and care of athletes. As an aside, it is interesting to speculate about the degree to which a preoccupation with obtaining the ideal nutritional supplement—an exogenous source of performance assistance—correlates with, or evolves into, a willingness to eventually seek other forms of exogenously administered performance "enhancers."

Those in the nutrition, sport medicine, and sport science communities should evaluate the nature, quality, and source of the advice that is currently being provided to athletes regarding diet and performance. A firm commitment to evidence-based practice and a more rigorous scrutiny of what is presented and published in the area of sport nutrition may arrest what seems to be a descent into a world of nostrums and nutritional pseudoscience. Current practices seem all the more skewed when one considers that while athletes and others are clamoring for supplements of various micro- or pseudonutrients, we face significant problems of major nutritional deficiencies in many sport settings. It is surprising to note that, when reviewing the declarations of medication and supplement use that accompany drug-testing samples, products such as iron, calcium, folate, and antioxidant vitamins are infrequently encountered—amidst a tidal wave of obscure and imaginatively named supplement products.

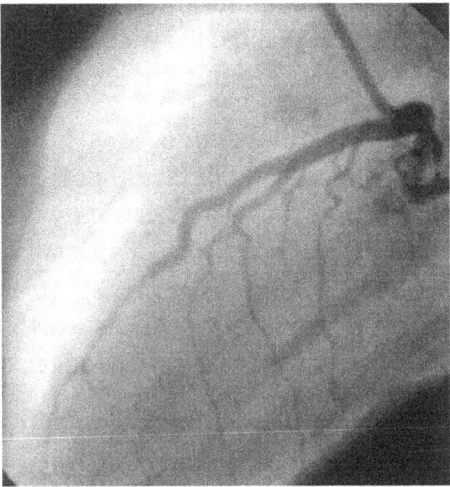

Marked spasm in the left anterior descending coronary artery of a young woman following the ingestion of a "natural" dietary product containing ephedrine. Cardiac arrest and prolonged resuscitation followed. The patient survived but experiences significant cerebral deficits.

Sport administrators need to ensure that athletes are being counseled by appropriately qualified nutrition professionals, and may wish to reconsider the wisdom of entering into sponsorship agreements with members of the nutritional supplement industry until such time as it becomes possible to verify the content, safety, quality, and labeling of its products. Sport physicians must be vigorous, and rigorous, in ensuring that the athletes entrusted to their care are in receipt of accurate information regarding their nutritional practices, and that they are not ingesting products that jeopardize their health or their status as competitors. Those involved in the development and administration of doping-control programs must continue to provide clear, unequivocal advice about the potential problems associated with supplement use while striving to be sensitive, imaginative, and credible in the delivery of those messages. Public authorities must be reminded of their responsibility to protect the public from misrepresentation and the dangers posed by hazardous products; the removal of ephedrine-containing products from the community and the regulation of dietary supplements would seem to be sensible steps. William Osler, many years ago, suggested "One of the first duties of the physician is to educate the masses not to take medicine." His advice, intended for a community in which "electric oil salesmen," carnival barkers, and traveling medicine shows exploited a gullible public, may have particular relevance for sport medicine practitioners today, when terms such as "herbal," "natural," "alternative," "complementary," and "supplement" may conceal a bizarre array of concoctions and compounds that are too often worthless and frequently harmful.

Doping in Sports

Doping has become a key and complex issue in the sports world, which deserves serious consideration, as specialists are still striving to understand how and why it happens, and how to prevent it. "Sensational" revelations in the press reflect the gravity of a worrying situation resonating in most sports disciplines.

Cases of doping compromise the credibility of performance in sport, the mediatized victories of some "arena heroes" becoming questionable and disputable. Nowadays some sporting disciplines seem to have managed to surpass the human limits and sometimes even the legal limits. The financial interests, the pressure to obtain better results, the media coverage of sports competitions and, last but not least, the human nature can explain this phenomenon.

It is clear that in some disciplines such as athletics or cycling, human performance cannot improve endlessly. Nowadays, sports are no longer just sports; as sport become an industry, a business, a reason for political or national pride, and these facts can only lead to breaking any rules to win. Sometimes, consciously, camouflaged, with a network of specialists behind or on their own, some athletes think "maybe they won't catch me"; because today sports mean sponsors, advertising contracts and money and for that some believe that any risk is worth taking. Even risks to their own health (often with huge and irreversible consequences) no longer matter.

The commercial side of a sporting event is also an important matter. If people like the event in the modern arena, then the commercial success of the sporting event is assured and the sponsors are satisfied and will finance future events, thus providing funds for the organizers to give substantial prizes for the athletes.

The doping phenomenon in sports is increasing and diversifying, as are the drugs used for doping. There is a permanent race among those who invent new doping methods and sports ethics organizations that are searching for more performant methods to detect them. Unfortunately, most of the times, those in the first category are always one step ahead.

Improving scientific procedures used to detect prohibited substances is of course a necessity and also a challenge. Stricter legislation with the involvement of authorities is required to prevent the spread, marketing and use of such substances. Resolute action is required to restore fair-play throughout the sports industry and last but not least, the ethics and fair-play education of young athletes.

Depending on the country's legislation, doping substances can be bought from pharmacies/supplement stores or, most commonly, from the black market. For a substance or performance improvement method to be classified as doping, it must meet at least two of the following three criteria: to improve performance, to present a hazard to the health of the athlete and to violate the spirit of sport. Other methods of improving performance such as blood transfusions are also included in the doping category.

Table: Banned substances both during and outside the competition.

Substances that have not been placed on the market	Retired drugs such as sibutramine	Designer substances: tetrahydro-gestrinone	Drugs used in veterinary medicine
Anabolic agents	Exogenous anabolic steroids: androstendiol and gestrinone	Endogenous anabolic steroids with exogenous administration: dihydrotestosterone, testosterone	Other anabolic agents: tibolone, zilpaterol, zeranol
Peptide hormones and growth factors	Erythropoiesis stimulating agents: erythropoietin, darboietin	Luteinizing hormone in men; choriogonadotrophin	Corticotrophins, Growth Hormones. Insulin-like growth factor 1 (IGF 1)
Beta 2 agonists	Salbutamol-1600 µg /24h	Formoterol 54 µg/ 24 h	Clenbuterol

Hormones and metabolic modulators	Aromatase inhibitors: aminoglutethimide	Metabolic mediators: insulin	-
Diuretics and other masking agents	Masking agents: glycerols, plasma substitutes	Diuretics: Acetazolamide, Furosemide, Indapamide	-
CNS stimulants	Nonspecific stimulants: amfepramone, fenfluramine	Specific stimulants: adrenaline, ephedrine, pseudoephedrine	-
Narcotics	Buprenorphine, fentanyl	Metadone, morphine	-
Cannabis extracts	Cannabis, hashish	Tetrahydrocannabinol	-
Corticosteroids	Cortizon, Hydrocortisone	Prednison, Metilprednisolone	-

Table: Prohibited methods.

Manipulation of blood and its components	Administration of products containing red blood cells in the circulatory system	Increasing the amount of oxygen or its transport
Physical and chemical handling	Altering the integrity and validity of the sample collected during anti-doping control	Intravenous infusions or injections of more than 50 mL for 6 hours
Genetically doping	Transfer of polymers of nucleic acids or their analogs	Use of normal or genetically modified cells

Substances which are not on the List of Prohibited Substances with Possible Doping Effect

One of the substances that are currently extensively studied for doping potential is paracetamol, a substance commonly used as an analgesic and antipyretic. It has been noticed that in the case of cyclists, the athletes performances have been improved. So if in the case of cyclists it can increase performance, by lowering body temperature; why couldn't it be used for athletes practicing marathon, or athletes who run the 5000 and 10000 meters distances?

Some herbal extracts were suspected to have doping effects, so the ginseng root was tested to detect possible performance enhancing effects, but according to studies conducted on athletes under the supervision of the IOC, no positive tests were observed. However, it is specified that due to contamination with other doping substances, the tests could be positive, due to which the nutraceuticals should be carefully checked prior to use, in order to prevent possible disqualification from competitions.

Studies have also been conducted to see whether NSAIDs, diclofenac and ibuprofen, both being non-selective COX non-steroidal anti-inflammatory drugs, could have an effect on the testosterone/glucuronidated epitestosterone ratio, but the results did not reveal any modification.

Substances that are not Forbidden but can Increase the Performance of the Athlete

L-carnitine is an endogenous compound, an aminoacid synthesized in the liver and kidneys from lysine and methionine, two essential amino acids. It can be found especially in food of animal origin, but also in plants such as soy beans, although in much smaller quantities. L-carnitine administration increases the HDL cholesterol fraction, and has neuroprotective properties in Alzheimer's disease. For athletes, the use of L-carnitine is based on the release of energy from lipids, saving a part of the glycogen from the muscles.

Arginine is a semi-essential amino acid that could be used to increase performance, because of NO (nitrogen monoxide) release and the formation of citrulline, NO having a vasodilatory effect. Athletes can use arginine to increase physical performance, muscle mass and also their resistance in high effort.

Hydroxycitric acid is a substance often found in food supplements and it can be extracted from species such as Hibiscus sabdariffa or Garcinia cambodgia. It was reported to be used for weight loss, but according to clinical trials, it does not have lipolysis effects.

Tyrosine is an essential amino acid that cannot be synthesized by the body and should be obtained through careful nutrition. It can also be used by athletes, with many beneficial effects such as reducing fat, controlling appetite. However, it is a dopamine precursor and so people with mental disorders or hyperthyroidism should not use it, as well as people with high risk of skin cancer because this amino acid leads to increased melatonin secretion. Another aspect to be considered is the period of the day when it is administered, because it is a precursor of adrenaline and noradrenaline that can cause stimulation of the nervous system.

Other amino acids or derivatives used to increase muscle strength and endurance are: carnozine, citrulline, glutamine, glycine and taurine. Taurine and carnosine have particular effects, being used as energizing substances.

Substances that are Dopant only if Certain Doses are Exceeded

There are some pharmacological classes of substances that have a quantitative upper limit, so can be used only in very small amounts, as: central nervous system stimulants such as caffeine and beta 2 selectives such as salbutamol or fenoterol.

Caffeine can be considered as a dopant substance due to its effects: slight bronchodilatation, which is beneficial for athletes participating in endurance races, and also increases the diuresis which can be beneficial if an athlete is doped and wants to rapidly eliminate the other drug in their body. Other effects of caffeine are: cerebral vasoconstrictor, increases gastric acidity and also the appetite. An athlete is considered doped when the urine concentration of caffeine is above 12 μg/mL.

Most beta 2 selective substances are banned from competitions, but there are exceptions such as salbutamol, which has a maximum inhalation dose of 1.6 mg/24h. If salbutamol is present in a concentration higher than 1000 ng/mL in urine the athlete can be considered as doped. Formoterol is a substance used in asthma and it is in the same category as salbutamol. The dose of inhaled formoterol is 54 μg/ 4h, and urine concentration should not exceed 40 ng/mL, otherwise the athlete is sanctioned according to the rules.

Specific central nervous system stimulants are substances that also have thresholds, ephedrine and methylefedrine are prohibited when the concentration reaches values higher than 10 μg/mL, pseudoephedrine is prohibited when concentrations are greater than 150 μg/mL. Adrenaline is not forbidden when used locally in nasal or ophthalmic administration.

Other substances that have a superior limit, that can lead to the elimination of the athlete from the competition are: bupropion, nicotine, pipradol, phenylephrine and phenylpropanolamine.

Substances Subject to a Monitoring Program

There are three classes of substances part of a monitoring program: central nervous system stimulants such as bupropion, nicotine, phenylephrine, phenylpropanolamine, sinephrine and pipradrol; narcotics: hydrocodone, tramadol, talpentadol; and glucocorticoids, banned in competition through all ways of administration. Also, telmisartan, a angiotensin II antagonist class on AT1 receptors and meldonium substance used in angina pectoris, can be included in the same category. Central nervous system stimulants as well as narcotics will not be used in competitions, while glucocorticoids, meldonium and telmisartan are banned both outside and in competitions.

Following are some of the substances and methods used for doping in sport:

Erythropoietin

Erythropoietin (EPO) is a peptide hormone that is produced naturally by the human body. EPO is released from the kidneys and acts on the bone marrow to stimulate red blood cell production.

By injecting EPO, athletes aim to increase the concentration of red blood cells and consequently their aerobic capacity.

EPO abuse can lead to serious health risks for athletes. It is well known that EPO, by thickening the blood, leads to an increased risk of several deadly diseases, such as heart disease, stroke, and cerebral or pulmonary embolism. EPO has been implicated in the deaths of several athletes.

Continuous Erythropoiesis Receptor Activator

Continuous Erythropoiesis Receptor Activator, or CERA, is a third-generation form of EPO. As opposed to earlier forms of the drug, CERA requires less frequent injection because it has an extended half-life.

Athletes may take CERA to increase oxygen-carrying capacity to boost endurance. It may also be used after training to encourage swifter recovery.

Anabolic Steroids

Anabolic steroids are drugs that resemble testosterone, a hormone which is produced in the testes of males and, to a much lesser extent, in the ovaries of females.

Because testosterone and related drugs affect muscle growth, raising their levels in the blood could help athletes to increase muscle size and strength. Athletes who use anabolic steroids also claim they reduce body fat and recovery time after injury.

Anabolic steroids can cause high blood pressure, acne, abnormalities in liver function, alterations in the menstrual cycle, decline in sperm production and impotence in men, kidney failure and heart disease. They can also make people more aggressive.

Examples of anabolic steroids include testosterone, stanozolol, boldenone, nandrolone and clostebol.

Human Growth Hormone

Human growth hormone (hGH)- also called somatotrophin or somatotrophic hormone - is a hormone that is naturally produced by the body. It is synthesized and secreted by cells in the anterior pituitary gland located at the base of the brain.

The major role of hGH in body growth is to stimulate the liver and other tissues to secrete insulin-like growth factor IGF-1. IGF-1 stimulates production of cartilage cells, resulting in bone growth and also plays a key role in muscle and organ growth. All of these can boost sporting performance.

Commonly reported side effects for hGH abuse are diabetes in prone individuals, worsening of heart diseases, muscle, joint and bone pain, hypertension and cardiac deficiency, abnormal growth of organs and accelerated osteoarthritis.

Diuretics

Diuretics can be used in a sport as a masking agent to prevent the detection of another banned substance.

As well as masking other drugs, diuretics can also help athletes lose weight, which they could use to their advantage in sports where they need to qualify in a particular weight category.

Examples of commonly used diuretics include furosemide, bendroflumethiazide and metolazone.

Synthetic Oxygen Carriers

Synthetic oxygen carriers, such as haemoglobin-based oxygen carriers (HBOCs) or perflurocarbons (PFCs), are purified proteins or chemicals that have the ability to carry oxygen.

They are useful for emergency therapeutic purposes when human blood is not available, the risk of blood infection is high or when there is not enough time to properly cross-match donated blood with a recipient.

The misuse of synthetic oxygen carriers for doping purposes carries the risk of cardiovascular disease in addition to serious side effects such as strokes, heart attacks and embolisms.

Blood Doping

There are two forms of blood doping. Autologous blood doping is the transfusion of one's own blood, which has been stored, refrigerated or frozen, until needed. Homologous blood doping is the transfusion of blood that has been taken from another person with the same blood type.

Although the use of blood transfusions for blood doping dates back several decades, experts say its recent resurgence is probably due to the introduction of efficient EPO detection methods. A test for homologous blood transfusions was implemented at the 2004 Olympic Games in Athens.

Insulin

Insulin enhances glucose uptake into the muscle and aids the formation and storage of muscle glycogen.

Athletes might use it for events that require high levels of endurance. There is also evidence that it is abused by dopers in conjunction with growth hormones or anabolic steroids to boost muscle growth.

Misuse of insulin can lead to very low blood sugar levels - a condition known as hypoglycaemia which can lead to the loss of cognitive function, seizures, unconsciousness, and in extreme cases can lead to brain damage of death.

Gene Doping

Advancements in gene therapy for medical reasons mean potential cheats might seek to undergo procedures to modify their genes to enhance their physical capabilities.

While it is not yet known whether it has ever been done in practice, gene doping could in theory be used to increase muscle growth, blood production, endurance, oxygen dispersal and pain perception.

Gene doping is defined by WADA as the transfer for nucleic acids or nucleic acid sequences, and the use of normal or genetically modified cells. There are currently no testing methods capable of detecting gene doping.

Doping Tests

Doping testing is an activity that is strictly specified in the International Standard for Testing and Investigations. Urine, blood or both are collected as test samples. Doping testing takes place both at competitions and outside of them.

Types

There are two types of doping tests: in-competition tests and out-of-competition tests. An athlete can be summoned to testing at any time and anywhere, either in their home country or abroad. The athlete is invited in person.

In-competition Tests

In-competition tests refer to doping tests performed in connection with a competition event. Unless otherwise specified in the rules of the international or another relevant antidoping organisation, this refers to a period starting 12 hours prior to the competition and ending at the end of the competition and the related collection of samples.

All known doping substances and methods and any manipulation of the sample are tested from samples collected in connection with competitions.

The athletes are drawn or ordered to undergo testing based on ranking, for example, or chosen for it as specified in the competition rules of the sport. The athletes can also be ordered to take the test by name in the in-competition tests.

In some sports, a record result cannot be officially approved until the athlete in question has produced a negative sample. After breaking a record, the athlete must attend the doping control in a manner provided by the rules of the sport.

Out-of-competition Tests

Targeted doping tests are also carried out outside of competitions. Out-of-competition samples are tested for non-approved substances, anabolic agents, peptide hormones, growth factors and similar substances, ß2-agonists, hormone and metabolism modulators, diuretics and other masking agents as well as all prohibited methods.

International sports federations may have rules of their own regarding the substances to be tested. It is the athletes responsibility to be aware of the relevant rules.

Athletes are chosen for out-of-competition tests in a targeted manner or by drawing the athletes to be tested during the training of a certain group or athletes on a camp.

Targeted tests are mainly carried out for testing pool and national team athletes. can, however, target any athlete bound by the antidoping code for testing, both in-competition and out-of-competition.

Out-of-competition tests also include follow-up tests made to clarify the results of previous tests and tests carried out during a period of ineligibility due to antidoping rule violations.

Sample Types

Doping tests consist of taking a urine sample or a blood sample or both. A blood sample does not replace a urine test, because it concerns primarily different substances and different methods.

Urine Tests

Doping control is most often carried out based on urine tests. The urine sample is used in analysing the use of prohibited substances and methods.

Blood Tests

Blood samples may be taken for identifying prohibited substances and methods, for screening or as a part of long-term monitoring in order to create an athlete's personal profile.

Blood samples are collected according to the instructions of the International Standard for Testing and Investigations. They are taken by a person who, in addition to training and authorisation, has vocational training in health care and is qualified to take blood samples. Blood tests are carried out, for example, in order to detect growth hormone and the use of various artificial substances and methods related to the manipulation of blood.

Athlete Biological Passport

Certain biological variables of an athlete will be monitored regularly throughout his/her athletic career. Changes in the athlete's profile may reveal the use of doping.

An athlete's individual profile, i.e. the so-called Athlete Biological Passport (ABP) system, is about monitoring selected biological variables (such as haemoglobin and haematocrit in the haematological profile and testosterone and epi-testosterone in the steroid profile) over an extended period of time. The results are used to create a profile which serves as an athlete's personal reference value range instead of population-based reference values used earlier.

The Athlete Biological Passport system can be used as a tool for targeting and scheduling testing. It can also be used for indirectly showing any use of doping agents or methods and therefore an antidoping rule violation.

5

Weight Management for Athletes

Weight management is important for improving athletic performance and helps in preventing the development of serious chronic diseases. A few of its aspects include body mass index, calorie restriction, weight gain and loss strategies, etc. All these weight management strategies for athletes have been carefully analyzed in this chapter.

Weight management is difficult for most individuals, as indicated by the high numbers of obesity around the world. Obesity has increased dramatically over the past decades. Unfortunately, this epidemic is not limited to adults but also to children in both globally and Cyprus. Developing a weight management plan is essential for everyone. Regarding to an athlete, weight management is an increasingly integral part, as consuming the right kind of food can lead them in success or failure. The special nutritional needs of athletes are depending on the sport. The most important priority for them is to establish a wellchosen nutrition program based on the type of the sport; the training load and the competitions needs. Health professionals and sport nutritionists need to understand dynamic energy balance and be prepared with effective and evidence-based dietary approaches to help athletes and active individuals achieve their body-weight goals. Therefore, the following review aiming to examine the most recent published data for weight-management both elite and recreational athletes of all ages, and to set out the most appropriate weight-management guidelines and dietary strategies to help them apply this knowledge to the practicalities of their own sport and individual situation.

Weight management is difficult for most individuals, as indicated by the high numbers of obesity around the world. Obesity is a global health epidemic characterized by excessive body fat accumulation. Individuals with body mass index (BMI) falling within 25-29.9kg/m² are indicated as overweight, whereas individuals with BMI at or above 30kg/m² are indicated as obese. Based on a study conducted in 2014, revealed that within four decades the global obesity in men has tripled, from 3.2% in 1975 to 10.8% in 2014. During the same period, obesity in women has more than doubled from 6.4% in 1975 to 14.9% in 2014.

Developing a weight management plan is essential for everyone. Proper nutrition plays an important role at peak performance, specifically when someone does exercise to keep fit, participate regularly in organized sports activities or training to reach the top level of the sport. With regard to an athlete, weight management is an increasingly integral part, as consuming the right kind of food can lead individually in the success or failure. If athletes combine serious restriction energy with a strong resistance and strength training program, then it can actually lead to metabolic changes. These two factors are extremely stressful for the athletes due to lose rapid body weight, also minimized their sports performance, and dangerous about their health.

The special nutritional needs of athletes are depending on the sport; whether they want to lose body fat or gaining and maintaining lean tissue. While some athletes appear to be naturally lean, with weight and body size well matched for their sport, others need to change their weight and body composition to be competitive. For instance, aesthetic sports e.g. rhythmic and artistic gymnastics, ice skating or dancing, weight division sports e.g. judo, or rowing gym sports e.g. aerobics, endurance sports e.g. long distance running are sports requiring low body-weight and body composition in order to considered an athlete as elite.

The most important priority for athletes is to establish a well-chosen nutrition program based on the type of the sport, body composition goals about the sport, also the training load and the competition needs. A proper athletic diet will provide adequate nutrients and energy to enhance adaptations from training, support optimal recovery with no food-related stress. It is known that heavy training, requires more nutrients and energy mainly in carbohydrate, protein and micronutrients (vitamins and minerals).

Health professionals and sport nutritionists need to understand dynamic energy balance and be prepared with effective and evidence-based dietary approaches to help athletes and active individuals achieve their body-weight goals.

Weight-control Behavior in Athletes

In general, most athletes who want to lose weight fall into two categories; those who are overweight or obese based on body-fat levels, and those who are already lean, but desire additional body fat loss. Some of these athletes fall into weight-sensitive (e.g., endurance athletes, ski jumping), weight-class (e.g., wrestling, judo), or aesthetically judged (e.g., gymnastics, figure skating) sports.

It is known that excess body fat decreasing athletic performance as well as could increase the risk of chronic diseases for athletes. One study found that 21% of first Division college football players were obese and had insulin resistance, while 9% had metabolic syndrome. Thus, for these athletes, weight loss could improve performance and prevent the development of serious chronic diseases.

Conversely, many elite and recreational athletes who have normal weight or low body weights, yet they still want to lose weight in order to improve their performance and to achieve a body shape for aesthetic reasons. Some of these individuals are young and still growing, which is the least desirable time to severely restrict energy intake while participating in high levels of exercise.

Restrict weight control and diet low in calories are particularly widespread in sports where focus in leanness (leanness-sports) or low body weight like aesthetic or endurance sports. One study showed that NCAA Division I athletes who competing in leanness sports, had significantly higher on the sub-score for Body Dissatisfaction and had lower mean desired body weight than those competing in non-leanness sports. This study was in line with Rosendahl et al. who compare leanness sports and non-leanness sports concluded that athletes competing in leanness sports scored higher for weight-control behaviour than those competing in non-leanness sports.

On the other hand, a study with 204 NCAA Division I, athletes of many sports types using the Questionnaire for Eating Disorder Diagnosis showed that over half of the athletes were not satisfied with their body weight. More of them wanted to lose weight (~5.9 kg), and also there was a weight fluctuation of more than 10% within a year of the athletes. They stated that the methods they used to reduce their body weight were exercise around 2 hours a day and the fasting or on a low calories diet.

Martinsen et al. had 606 elite athletes from 50 different sports types who showed similar frequencies of pathogenic weight-control methods like vomiting, laxatives, diuretics and diet pills. It seemed that between female and male athletes, the female athletes used more these pathogenic weight-control methods. When looking at weight concerns, the 24% of the female athletes and 7.5% of the male athletes were presently on a diet and have been on a diet at least three times before due to this reason.

In addition, for athletes in aesthetic sports like figure skaters, synchronized swimmers, gymnasts, maintaining a low body weight over a competitive season without injury or illness or the use of extreme weight-control methods is also a challenge. In a study of psychosocial correlates of bulimic symptoms were participated 280 NCAA Division I female gymnasts and 134 NCAA Division I female swimmers/divers showed that the level of body dissatisfaction, as well as restrictive eating, was related to the amount of experienced pressure from teammates and coaches.

Other study showed that there was no difference about the weight-concerns between the synchronized swimmers and other "non-weight dependent sports types" such as basketball, volleyball, soccer.

However, it seemed that it can be difficult to manage safe weight loss in athletes who need to meet a designated weight on competition day, like lightweight rowers, jockeys, or wrestlers. These individuals typically weight cycle, with their weight fluctuating dramatically between the competitive and off seasons.

Looking at weight-dependent sports, three studies described methods of rapid weight-control amongst judo athletes and one study for Taekwondo. The first one where was among elite male and female judo athletes showed that 86% have reduced body weight rapidly before the competition (around 2-5%), with some athletes losing up to 10% ten times or more in their careers. The fluctuation of weight was confirmed with a study of Rouveix et al. which showed that quick weight reduction is an inherent part of the judo athletes. Also, 70% of the athletes seemed that lost more than 2.8 kg during a season, with the methods of excessive exercises or limit the food and fluids consumption.

Moreover, in a cross-sectional study of Berkovich et al. were used 108 male athletes from local judo teams. Rapid Weight Loss (RWL) was practiced by 80% of the athletes before competition, beginning at an average age of 12.5 ± 2.2 years with the highest prevalence (~94%) in the oldest group of judoka (16–17.9 years). Precompetition weight loss duration was 8 ± 5.4 days, with an average weight reduction of 1.5 ± 1.1 kg. The number of weight loss efforts per athlete in the past season was 2.8 ± 2.2. RWL was achieved by increased physical activity (82.6%), skipped meals (56.3%), or fasting at least once (47%). Two-thirds of the athletes indicated that they experienced pressure from their coaches and were the most influential figure in their decision to lose weight before competition. These athletes used the methods which compromised nutritional status, diminished physical performance and impaired growth and development. These methods can potentially lead to significant health risks. A key priority for the persons who guide young adults in weight loss for competitive sports is to have the knowledge and understanding to make safe recommendations and appropriate decisions about achieving specific and healthy weight goals.

Moreover, Sandos et al. investigated the prevalence, magnitude, and methods of quick weight loss among 72 male and 44 female Taekwondo athletes from all competitive levels. The results from the given questionnaires have shown that among the male athletes, 77.4% of the regional/state level and 75.6% of the national/international athletes declared to have reduced weight to compete in lighter weight categories. Among women, 88.9% of regional/state level and 88.6% of national/international level were using rapid weight loss strategies. Athletes reported to usually lose around 3% of their body weight, with some athletes reaching around 7% of their body weight. The methods used to achieve weight loss are potentially dangerous for health and had no difference between sexes.

Four methods were more frequently used by men athletes in higher competitive levels as compared to lower levels, as follows: skipping meals, fasting, restricting fluids and spitting. Taekwondo athletes lost around 3% of their body mass, using the health-dangerous methods. Although no difference was found between sexes, while lower level athletes typically skip meals, fast, restrict fluids and spitting. Considering that these healththreating methods are more commonly used by lower level athletes, specific education programs should be directed to them.

Another study investigated the methods adopted to reduce body mass (BM) in competitive athletes from the grappling (judo, jujitsu) and striking (karate and taekwondo) combat sports in Brazil. A standardized questionnaire was used with objective questions self-administered to 580 athletes. Regardless of the sport, 60% of the athletes reported using a method of RWL via increased energy expenditure. Strikers tend to begin reducing BM during adolescence. Furthermore, 50% of the sample used saunas and plastic clothing, and only 26.1% received advice from a nutritionist. In addition, a high percentage of athletes use unapproved or prohibited methods such as diuretics, saunas, and plastic clothing. Few athletes are naturally light weight enough for these types of competitive sports, thus weight loss will be required the weeks or days prior to competition.

According to a research, depending on the sport, the weight of an athlete during the competitive season is usually lower than the weight in off season. As a result of this, most of the athletes restricting their energy intake in order to achieve their competitive weight and they often gain the lost-weight back during the off season. The ultimate goal for everyone and for athletes as well, is to develop healthy eating habits so as to achieve a healthy body weight that they can maintain for most of the year. In that way, athletes reducing the amount of weight that need to be lost for competition. The same research supported that for some sports, losing high amount of weight - for the needs of the competitive season - is not healthy for most athletes. Moreover, Manore continued by saying that the key priority for each athlete is to make sure that their goal-weight is realistic and will not cause any health issues and increase the risk of injuries.

Taking into consideration their ages as well as the level of their physical development are some ways that can help the athlete identify whether the weight they are trying to achieve is realistic. Sport dietitians are the health professionals should monitor athletes to help them reach their body-weight goals and to assure they are maintaining healthy eating habits.

While thinking of dietary strategies, expect to be analyzed evidence-based diet and lifestyle guidelines for athletes who are having a weight-specific goal; whether they are interested in losing weight, maintaining lean tissue and preventing weight regain.

Energy Restriction Approaches

The approach for restricting energy intake combined with an intense endurance and strength-training program can actually increase metabolic adaptations that slow weight loss and diminish the additive effects of these two factors on weight loss. But, this approach should be avoided because athletes are leading in a number of other negative performance and health consequences. For example, decreased athletic performance effects due to decreased muscle strength, glycogen stores, concentration, coordination and training responses, and increased irritability. Also, increased negative health consequences (injury due to fatigue, loss of lean tissue, poor nutrient intakes, etc), increased risk of disordered eating behaviors, dehydration, and emotional distress due to hunger, fatigue, and stress.

It is important to remember that with negative energy balance, lean, fit individuals can quickly lose lean tissue if energy is restricted too dramatically. For instance, one study placed active military personnel (BMI $25 \pm 1 \text{ kg/m}^2$) on a 40 % energyrestricted diet for 30 days, while being fed the recommended dietary allowance (RDA) for protein (0.8 g/kg/body weight). Of the 3.3 kg lost during this time (4.2 % body weight), 58 % was lean tissue (1.9 kg). In contrast, when they placed sedentary overweight individuals (BMI 27.8 kg/m^2) on a 25 % energy-restriction diet for 3 months, they lost 6 kg, with only 33 % coming from lean tissue (2 kg). Furthermore, Garthe et al. showed that the athletes who had slower, and more logical weight loss around 0.7 % loss of body weight per week helped maintain lean tissue while improving strength gains compared with more severe weight loss (1.4 % weight loss/week).

Therefore, for the athletes who already have a training, it is preferable to moderately restrict energy intake (e.g., 500–700 kcal/day) and take longer to reach the weight loss goal (0.50-1 kg /week). This approach also allows the time required to adapt to new dietary habits while making sure adequate energy is available for exercise training.

Timing of Food Consumption during Training and throughout the Day

Timing of food intake around exercise training and spreading food intake throughout the day is a key priority for the athlete. This approach ensures that the body has the nutrients and energy needed for the specific exercise and the building and repairing of lean tissue. Furthermore, may delay hunger and as an extension of this may prevent the athlete from consuming foods or beverages not included in their diet plan.

It is evidence-based that when athletes are concerned about their weight -particularly female athletes- they usually skipping meals, mainly breakfast. Recent study of Erdman reported that 98% of elite Canadian male athletes consumed breakfast, while Shriver et al. at the same year found that only 23% of elite college female athletes consumed breakfast. The majority of the athletes in the second study reported their diets to be poor, most of the calories were consuming at dinner and they found it difficult to maintain their weight. Those eating habits may be a result of the idea that skipping breakfast will help in reducing caloric intake, therefore the overall weight.

Focusing on the athlete, breakfast constitutes the most important meal of the day, mainly due to the fact that it can provide carbohydrates needed to help replenish lost glycogen after an overnight fast and provide the appropriate fuel for exercise.

For those who participate in an early-morning workout, eating a light pre-workout snack and a nutritious post-workout breakfast will assure the adequate nutrients have been lost during exercise particularly carbohydrate and protein. In a research examined the importance of breakfast for athletes, it was found that during moderate training weeks, breakfast provided 21% of the daily carbohydrate intake for junior elite triathletes, while during high intensity training weeks, breakfast provided 28% of their daily carbohydrate intake. Therefore, skipping breakfast would lower total daily carbohydrate intake, thus affecting exercise performance.

Post-workout meal is crucial as well, since it provides to the athlete all the necessary nutrients for the replenishment of lost glycogen, and also building and repairing their lean tissue. An appropriate post-workout meal should compose of foods high in fluids for rehydration and carbohydrates in the form of low energy dense foods, such as whole fruits and vegetables and whole grains. Sport dietitians should monitor athletes so as to ensure they develop healthy eating habits and prepare the most appropriate diet plan according to the individual needs. Overall, the use of low energy dense diet plan is the most effective way for refueling during training periods, while during competitive periods there is a need for higher energy dense foods if glycogen replacement needs to occur in less than 24 hours.

Body Mass Index

Body mass index (BMI) is a value derived from the mass (weight) and height of a person. The BMI is defined as the body mass divided by the square of the body height, and is universally expressed in units of kg/m^2, resulting from mass in kilograms and height in metres.

The BMI may be determined using a table or chart which displays BMI as a function of mass and height using contour lines or colours for different BMI categories, and which may use other units of measurement (converted to metric units for the calculation).

The BMI is a convenient rule of thumb used to broadly categorize a person as underweight, normal weight, overweight, or obese based on tissue mass (muscle, fat, and bone) and height. That categorization is the subject of some debate about where on the BMI scale the dividing lines between categories should be placed. Commonly accepted BMI ranges are underweight: under 18.5 kg/m^2, normal weight: 18.5 to 25, overweight: 25 to 30, obese: over 30.

BMIs under 20.0 and over 25.0 have been associated with higher all-causes mortality, with the risk increasing with distance from the 20.0–25.0 range.

The BMI is universally expressed in kg/m², resulting from mass in kilograms and height in metres. If pounds and inches are used, a conversion factor of 703 (kg/m²)/(lb/in²) must be applied. When the term BMI is used informally, the units are usually omitted.

$$BMI = \frac{mass_{kg}}{height_m^2} = \frac{mass_{lb}}{height_{in}^2} \times 703$$

BMI provides a simple numeric measure of a person's *thickness* or *thinness*, allowing health professionals to discuss weight problems more objectively with their patients. BMI was designed to be used as a simple means of classifying average sedentary (physically inactive) populations, with an average body composition. For such individuals, the value recommendations as of 2014 are as follows: a BMI from 18.5 up to 25 kg/m² may indicate optimal weight, a BMI lower than 18.5 suggests the person is underweight, a number from 25 up to 30 may indicate the person is overweight, and a number from 30 upwards suggests the person is obese. Lean male athletes often have a high muscle-to-fat ratio and therefore a BMI that is misleadingly high relative to their body-fat percentage.

Scalability

BMI is proportional to the mass and inversely proportional to the square of the height. So, if all body dimensions double, and mass scales naturally with the cube of the height, then BMI doubles instead of remaining the same. This results in taller people having a reported BMI that is uncharacteristically high, compared to their actual body fat levels. In comparison, the Ponderal index is based on the natural scaling of mass with the third power of the height.

However, many taller people are not just "scaled up" short people but tend to have narrower frames in proportion to their height. Carl Lavie has written that, "The B.M.I. tables are excellent for identifying obesity and body fat in large populations, but they are far less reliable for determining fatness in individuals."

Categories

A frequent use of the BMI is to assess how far an individual's body weight departs from what is normal or desirable for a person's height. The weight excess or deficiency may, in part, be accounted for by body fat (adipose tissue) although other factors such as muscularity also affect BMI significantly.

The WHO regards a BMI of less than 18.5 as underweight and may indicate malnutrition, an eating disorder, or other health problems, while a BMI equal to or greater than 25 is considered overweight and above 30 is considered obese. These ranges of BMI values are valid only as statistical categories.

Category	BMI (kg/m²)		BMI Prime	
	from	to	from	to
Very severely underweight		15		0.60
Severely underweight	15	16	0.60	0.64
Underweight	16	18.5	0.64	0.74
Normal (healthy weight)	18.5	25	0.74	1.0

Overweight	25	30	1.0	1.2
Obese Class I (Moderately obese)	30	35	1.2	1.4
Obese Class II (Severely obese)	35	40	1.4	1.6
Obese Class III (Very severely obese)	40	45	1.6	1.8
Obese Class IV (Morbidly obese)	45	50	1.8	2
Obese Class V (Super obese)	50	60	2	2.4
Obese Class VI (Hyper obese)	60		2.4	

Body Mass Index values for males and females aged 20 and over, and selected percentiles by age

Age	Percentile								
	5th	10th	15th	25th	50th	75th	85th	90th	95th
	Men BMI (kg/m^2)								
20 years and over (total)	20.7	22.2	23.0	24.6	27.7	31.6	34.0	36.1	39.8
20–29 years	19.3	20.5	21.2	22.5	25.5	30.5	33.1	35.1	39.2
30–39 years	21.1	22.4	23.3	24.8	27.5	31.9	35.1	36.5	39.3
40–49 years	21.9	23.4	24.3	25.7	28.5	31.9	34.4	36.5	40.0
50–59 years	21.6	22.7	23.6	25.4	28.3	32.0	34.0	35.2	40.3
60–69 years	21.6	22.7	23.6	25.3	28.0	32.4	35.3	36.9	41.2
70–79 years	21.5	23.2	23.9	25.4	27.8	30.9	33.1	34.9	38.9
80 years and over	20.0	21.5	22.5	24.1	26.3	29.0	31.1	32.3	33.8
Age	Women BMI (kg/m^2)								
20 years and over (total)	19.6	21.0	22.0	23.6	27.7	33.2	36.5	39.3	43.3
20–29 years	18.6	19.8	20.7	21.9	25.6	31.8	36.0	38.9	42.0
30–39 years	19.8	21.1	22.0	23.3	27.6	33.1	36.6	40.0	44.7
40–49 years	20.0	21.5	22.5	23.7	28.1	33.4	37.0	39.6	44.5
50–59 years	19.9	21.5	22.2	24.5	28.6	34.4	38.3	40.7	45.2
60–69 years	20.0	21.7	23.0	24.5	28.9	33.4	36.1	38.7	41.8
70–79 years	20.5	22.1	22.9	24.6	28.3	33.4	36.5	39.1	42.9
80 years and over	19.3	20.4	21.3	23.3	26.1	29.7	30.9	32.8	35.2

Consequences of Elevated Level in Adults

The BMI ranges are based on the relationship between body weight and disease and death. Overweight and obese individuals are at an increased risk for the following diseases:

- Coronary artery disease.

- Dyslipidemia.

- Type 2 diabetes.

- Gallbladder disease.

- Hypertension.

- Osteoarthritis.

- Sleep apnea.

- Stroke.

- At least 10 cancers, including endometrial, breast, and colon cancer.

- Epidural lipomatosis.

Among people who have never smoked, overweight/obesity is associated with 51% increase in mortality compared with people who have always been a normal weight.

Applications

Public Health

The BMI is generally used as a means of correlation between groups related by general mass and can serve as a vague means of estimating adiposity. The duality of the BMI is that, while it is easy to use as a general calculation, it is limited as to how accurate and pertinent the data obtained from it can be. Generally, the index is suitable for recognizing trends within sedentary or overweight individuals because there is a smaller margin of error. The BMI has been used by the WHO as the standard for recording obesity statistics since the early 1980s.

This general correlation is particularly useful for consensus data regarding obesity or various other conditions because it can be used to build a semi-accurate representation from which a solution can be stipulated, or the RDA for a group can be calculated. Similarly, this is becoming more and more pertinent to the growth of children, due to the fact that the majority of children are sedentary. Cross-sectional studies indicated that sedentary people can decrease BMI by becoming more physically active. Smaller effects are seen in prospective cohort studies which lend to support active mobility as a means to prevent a further increase in BMI.

Clinical Practice

BMI categories are generally regarded as a satisfactory tool for measuring whether sedentary individuals are underweight, overweight, or obese with various exceptions, such as: athletes, children, the elderly, and the infirm. Also, the growth of a child is documented against a BMI-measured growth chart. Obesity trends can then be calculated from the difference between the child's BMI and the BMI on the chart. In the United States, BMI is also used as a measure of underweight, owing to advocacy on behalf of those with eating disorders, such as anorexia nervosa and bulimia nervosa.

Legislation

In France, Italy, and Spain, legislation has been introduced banning the usage of fashion show models having a BMI below 18. In Israel, a BMI below 18.5 is banned. This is done to fight anorexia among models and people interested in fashion.

Limitations

The medical establishment and statistical community have both highlighted the limitations of BMI.

Scaling

The exponent in the denominator of the formula for BMI is arbitrary. The BMI depends upon weight and the *square* of height. Since mass increases to the *third power* of linear dimensions, taller individuals with exactly the same body shape and relative composition have a larger BMI.

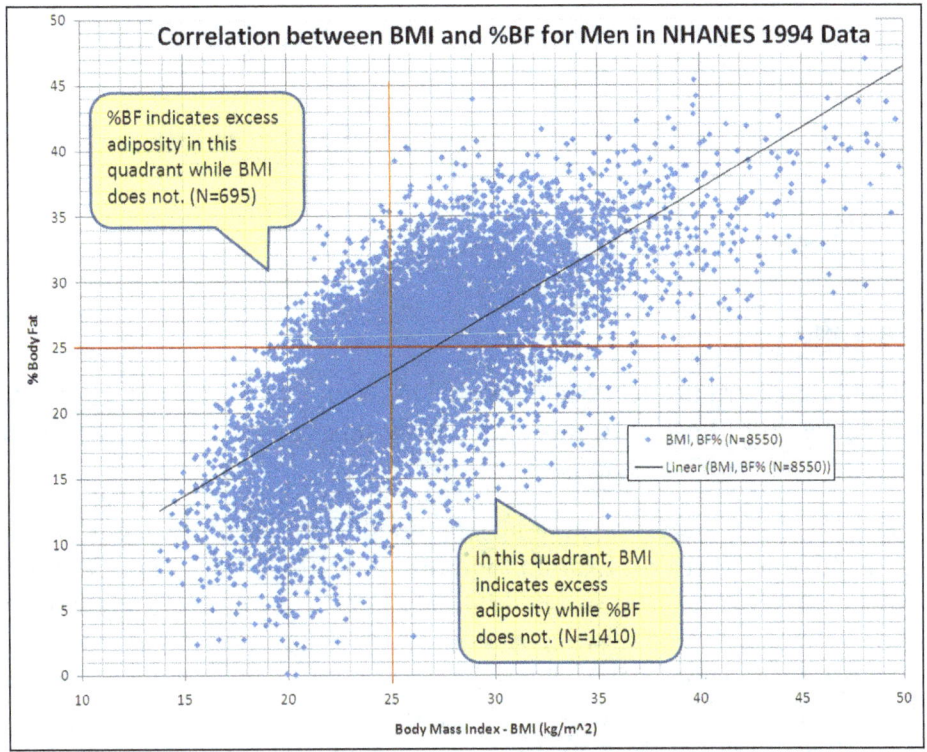

This graph shows the correlation between body mass index (BMI) and percent body fat (%BF) for 8550 men.

According to mathematician Nick Trefethen, "BMI divides the weight by too large a number for short people and too small a number for tall people. So short people are misled into thinking that they are thinner than they are, and tall people are misled into thinking they are fatter."

For US adults, exponent estimates range from 1.92 to 1.96 for males and from 1.45 to 1.95 for females.

Physical Characteristics

The BMI overestimates roughly 10% for a large (or tall) frame and underestimates roughly 10% for a smaller frame (short stature). In other words, persons with small frames would be carrying more fat than optimal, but their BMI indicates that they are *normal*. Conversely, large framed (or tall) individuals may be quite healthy, with a fairly low body fat percentage, but be classified as *overweight* by BMI.

For example, a height/weight chart may say the ideal weight (BMI 21.5) for a man 5 ft 10 in (178 cm) is 150 pounds (68 kg). But if that man has a slender build (small frame), he may be overweight at 150 pounds (68 kg) and should reduce by 10%, to roughly 135 pounds (61 kg) (BMI 19.4). In the reverse, the man with a larger frame and more solid build should increase by 10%, to roughly 165 pounds (75 kg) (BMI 23.7). If one teeters on the edge of small/medium or medium/large, common sense should be used in calculating one's ideal weight. However, falling into one's ideal weight range for height and build is still not as accurate in determining health risk factors as waist-to-height ratio and actual body fat percentage.

Accurate frame size calculators use several measurements (wrist circumference, elbow width, neck circumference and others) to determine what category an individual falls into for a given height. The BMI also fails to take into account loss of height through aging. In this situation, BMI will increase without any corresponding increase in weight.

A new formula, that accounts for the distortions of BMI at high and low heights, has been suggested:

$$\text{BMI} = 1.3 \times \frac{\text{mass}_{\text{kg}}}{\text{height}_{\text{m}}^{2.5}}$$

Muscle versus Fat

Assumptions about the distribution between muscle mass and fat mass are inexact. BMI generally overestimates adiposity on those with more lean body mass (e.g., athletes) and underestimates excess adiposity on those with less lean body mass.

A study in June 2008 by Romero-Corral et al. examined 13,601 subjects from the United States' third National Health and Nutrition Examination Survey (NHANES III) and found that BMI-defined obesity (BMI > 30) was present in 21% of men and 31% of women. Body fat-defined obesity was found in 50% of men and 62% of women. While BMI-defined obesity showed high specificity (95% for men and 99% for women), BMI showed poor sensitivity (36% for men and 49% for women). In other words, BMI is better at determining a person is not obese than it is at determining a person is obese. Despite this undercounting of obesity by BMI, BMI values in the intermediate BMI range of 20–30 were found to be associated with a wide range of body fat percentages. For men with a BMI of 25, about 20% have a body fat percentage below 20% and about 10% have body fat percentage above 30%.

BMI is particularly inaccurate for people who are very fit or athletic, as their high muscle mass can classify them in the *overweight* category by BMI, even though their body fat percentages frequently fall in the 10–15% category, which is below that of a more sedentary person of average build who has a *normal* BMI number. For example, the BMI of bodybuilder and eight-time Mr. Olympia Ronnie Coleman was 41.8 at his peak physical condition, which would be considered morbidly obese. Body composition for athletes is often better calculated using measures of body fat, as determined by such techniques as skinfold measurements or underwater weighing and the limitations of manual measurement have also led to new, alternative methods to measure obesity, such as the body volume index.

Variation in Definitions of Categories

It is not clear where on the BMI scale the threshold for *overweight* and *obese* should be set. Because of this the standards have varied over the past few decades. Between 1980 and 2000 the U.S. Dietary Guidelines have defined overweight at a variety of levels ranging from a BMI of 24.9 to 27.1. In 1985 the National Institutes of Health (NIH) consensus conference recommended that overweight BMI be set at a BMI of 27.8 for men and 27.3 for women.

In 1998 a NIH report concluded that a BMI over 25 is overweight and a BMI over 30 is obese. In the 1990s the World Health Organization (WHO) decided that a BMI of 25 to 30 should be considered overweight and a BMI over 30 is obese, the standards the NIH set. This became the definitive guide for determining if someone is overweight.

The current WHO and NIH ranges of normal weights are proved to be associated with decreased risks of some diseases such as diabetes type II; however using the same range of BMI for men and women is considered arbitrary, and makes the definition of underweight quite unsuitable for men.

One study found that the vast majority of people labelled 'overweight' and 'obese' according to current definitions do not in fact face any meaningful increased risk for early death. In a quantitative analysis of a number of studies, involving more than 600,000 men and women, the lowest mortality rates were found for people with BMIs between 23 and 29; most of the 25–30 range considered 'overweight' was not associated with higher risk.

Relationship to Health

A study in 2005 showed that overweight people had a death rate similar to normal weight people as defined by BMI, while underweight and obese people had a higher death rate.

A study in 2009 involving 900,000 adults showed that overweight and underweight people both had a mortality rate higher than normal weight people as defined by BMI. The optimal BMI was found to be in the range of 22.5–25. High BMI is associated with type 2 diabetes only in persons with high serum gamma-glutamyl transpeptidase.

In an analysis of 40 studies involving 250,000 people, patients with coronary artery disease with normal BMIs were at higher risk of death from cardiovascular disease than people whose BMIs put them in the overweight range (BMI 25–29.9).

One study found that BMI had a good general correlation with body fat percentage, and noted that obesity has overtaken smoking as the world's number one cause of death. But it also notes that in the study 50% of men and 62% of women were obese according to body fat defined obesity, while only 21% of men and 31% of women were obese according to BMI, meaning that BMI was found to underestimate the number of obese subjects.

A 2010 study that followed 11,000 subjects for up to eight years concluded that BMI is not a good measure for the risk of heart attack, stroke or death. A better measure was found to be the waist-to-height ratio. A 2011 study that followed 60,000 participants for up to 13 years found that waist–hip ratio was a better predictor of ischaemic heart disease mortality.

Alternatives

BMI Prime

BMI Prime, a modification of the BMI system, is the ratio of actual BMI to upper limit optimal BMI (currently defined at 25 kg/m²), i.e., the actual BMI expressed as a proportion of upper limit optimal. The ratio of actual body weight to body weight for upper limit optimal BMI (25 kg/m²) is equal to BMI Prime. BMI Prime is a dimensionless number independent of units. Individuals with BMI Prime less than 0.74 are underweight; those with between 0.74 and 1.00 have optimal weight; and those at 1.00 or greater are overweight. BMI Prime is useful clinically because it shows by what ratio (e.g. 1.36) or percentage (e.g. 136%, or 36% above) a person deviates from the maximum optimal BMI.

For instance, a person with BMI 34 kg/m² has a BMI Prime of 34/25 = 1.36, and is 36% over their upper mass limit. In South East Asian and South Chinese populations. BMI Prime should be calculated using an upper limit BMI of 23 in the denominator instead of 25. BMI Prime allows easy comparison between populations whose upper-limit optimal BMI values differ.

Waist Circumference

Waist circumference is a good indicator of visceral fat, which poses more health risks than fat elsewhere. According to the U.S. National Institutes of Health (NIH), waist circumference in excess of 102 centimetres (40 in) for men and 88 centimetres (35 in) for (non-pregnant) women, is considered to imply a high risk for type 2 diabetes, dyslipidemia, hypertension, and CVD. Waist circumference can be a better indicator of obesity-related disease risk than BMI. For example, this is the case in populations of Asian descent and older people. 94 centimetres (37 in) for men and 80 centimetres (31 in) for women has been stated to pose "higher risk", with the NIH figures "even higher".

Waist-to-hip circumference ratio has also been used, but has been found to be no better than waist circumference alone, and more complicated to measure.

A related indicator is waist circumference divided by height. The values indicating increased risk are: greater than 0.5 for people under 40 years of age, 0.5 to 0.6 for people aged 40–50, and greater than 0.6 for people over 50 years of age.

Surface-based Body Shape Index

The Surface-based Body Shape Index (SBSI) is far more rigorous and is based upon four key measurements: the body surface area (BSA), vertical trunk circumference (VTC), waist circumference (WC) and height (H). Study on 11,808 subjects from the National Health and Human Nutrition Examination Surveys (NHANES) 1999–2004, showed that SBSI outperformed BMI, waist circumference, and A Body Shape Index (ABSI), an alternative to BMI.

$$SBSI = \frac{(H^{7/4})(WC^{5/6})}{BSA\ VTC}$$

A simplified, dimensionless form of SBSI, known as SBSI*, has also been developed.

$$SBSI^* = \frac{(H^2)(WC)}{BSA\ VTC}$$

Modified Body Mass Index

Within some medical contexts, such as familial amyloid polyneuropathy, serum albumin is factored in to produce a modified body mass index (mBMI). The mBMI can be obtained by multiplying the BMI by serum albumin, in grams per litre.

Sport Performance and Body Composition

All fitness components depend on body composition to some extent. An increase in lean body mass contributes to strength and power development. Strength and power are related to muscle size. Thus, an increase in lean body mass enables the athlete to generate more force in a specific period of time. A sufficient level of lean body mass also contributes to speed, quickness, and agility performance (in the development of force applied to the ground for maximal acceleration and deceleration). Reduced nonessential body fat contributes to muscular and cardiorespiratory endurance, speed, and agility development. Additional weight (in the form of nonessential fat) provides greater resistance to athletic motion thereby forcing the athlete to increase the muscle force of contraction per given workload. The additional body fat can limit endurance, balance, coordination, and movement capacity. Joint range of motion can be negatively affected by excessive body mass and fat as well, and mass can form a physical barrier to joint movement in a complete range of motion. Thus, athletes competing in sports that require high levels of flexibility benefit from having low levels of body fat.

The demands of the sport require that athletes maintain standard levels of body composition. Some sports require athletes to be large in stature, mass, or both, whereas some athletes prosper when they are small in stature. For example, linemen in American football and heavyweight wrestlers need high levels of body mass. Although lean body mass is ideal, these athletes can benefit from mass increases in either form (fat included). Greater mass provides these athletes with more inertia, enabling them to play their positions with greater stability provided speed and agility are not compromised. Strength and power athletes such as American football players, wrestlers, and other combat athletes; powerlifters; bodybuilders; weightlifters; and track and field throwers benefit greatly from high levels of lean body mass. Endurance athletes such as distance runners, cyclists, and triathletes benefit greatly from having low percent body fat. Athletes such as gymnasts, wrestlers, high jumpers, pole vaulters, boxers, mixed martial artists, and weightlifters benefit greatly from having a high strength-to-mass (and power-to-mass) ratio. Training to maximize strength and power while minimizing changes in body mass (and keeping body fat low) is of great value to these sports. Gymnasts, pole vaulters, and high jumpers have to overcome their body weights to obtain athletic success. Thus, minimizing changes in mass enables greater flight height, time, and aerial athleticism.

Wrestlers, boxers, mixed martial artists, powerlifters, and weightlifters compete in weight classes. Because higher weight classes may denote more difficult competition, these athletes benefit from improving strength and power while maintaining their normal weight class. Athletes such as baseball and softball players benefit from increased lean body mass and reduced body fat. The additional lean mass can assist in power, speed, and agility, and keeping body fat low assists with endurance, quickness, speed, and agility as well (for performing skills such as throwing, hitting, fielding, and base running).

Basketball and soccer are two of several combination anaerobic and aerobic sports in which athletes need power, speed, quickness, agility, and strength yet also moderate to high levels of aerobic fitness. Athletes from both of these sports benefit from having low body fat while maintaining or increasing lean body mass. Although some athletes can tolerate higher levels of body mass and perhaps percent body fat, it is generally recommended that data obtained from frequent body composition measurements be used to develop training plans aimed at reducing body fat while maintaining or increasing lean body mass.

Obesity

Maintaining appropriate body weight is important for athletic performance. Body mass index (BMI) is commonly used to classify an individual's body weight. However, in the case of athletes, who may have a high body weight due to higher lean body mass, BMI may lead to misclassification of the athlete as overweight or obese. Thus, both BMI and body composition assessment should be conducted before determining if an athlete is overweight or obese. Body weight goals of athletes should be determined for each athlete, based on the requirements of the sport, the athlete's body size and shape, and in consultation with the athlete, coaches, and trainers. Safe weight loss goals should be established on an individual basis. Athletes, coaches, and trainers should work closely with individuals who have training in nutrition (registered dietitians) to set appropriate weight goals and to develop weight management protocols that promote healthy eating.

Obesity is currently a major epidemic in the Western world and is projected to be the leading cause of death in the United States, surpassing tobacco, by the year 2005. Poor diet and physical inactivity, major players in the obesity epidemic, account for 400,000 deaths (16.6% of total deaths), compared with 300,000 deaths (14% of total deaths) a decade ago.

Despite a national health objective to decrease the prevalence of obesity in adults to less than 15% of the population by 2010, overweight and obesity are continuing to rise among adults and children. Age-adjusted prevalence of obesity was 30.5% in 1999-2000 compared with 22.9% in the National Health and Nutrition Examination Survey (NHANES) III. The prevalence of overweight also increased during this period from 55.9% to 64.5%. These increases in the prevalence of overweight and obesity have been observed to occur in all ethnic and age groups, with little differences across the sexes. Additionally, among children and adolescents aged 6 to 19 years, 15% were found to be overweight and 10% of children between the ages of2 and 5 are now over weight.

Similar to the general population, body weights of certain groups of athletes have also been creeping upward. For example, on average collegiate football linemen weighed 220 lbs in 1963, compared with 331 lbs in 2003. These changes in body weight are reflective not only of the changing requirements of the various sports, and the impact of body size on performance, but also demands of other environmental factors, such as increase in fast food consumption, larger portion sizes, hectic schedules, and traveling away for competitions. Heitmann and Carby noted weight differences within each sex group for the same body height, which might be reflective of the genetic and environmental factors determining athlete's body weight.

Body Mass Index Classification of Athletes Body Weight

Using the BMI classifications, some athletes may be wrongly classified as overweight and obese, whereas in fact the excess weight may be due to increased muscle mass rather than increased body fat mass. Therefore, relying on the BMI to classify an athlete's weight may be inappropriate under certain conditions. Instead, a body composition analysis maybe more beneficial in determining an athlete's body weight status, given that increased body fat is associated with risk of certain chronic diseases as opposed to increased muscle mass. Furthermore, increased muscle mass, that is, lean body mass, has performance-enhancing effects, whereas increased body fat has a negative impact on performance, except under certain conditions, such as with Sumo wrestlers and football linemen, where blocking ability, rather than aerobic capacity and power, are beneficial in achieving the goals of the sport. Thus, in athletes, BMI could be useful as an initial assessment of the athlete's weight status, especially in sports in which body image and aesthetics are important to performance, such as gymnastics and figure skating. Athletes in these sports, especially women, typically have BMis in the range of 20 to 22, which they consider to be overweight, which is an unhealthy attitude. Thus, determination of BMI, along with body composition assessment, under these circumstances can help dissuade unrealistic body weight expectations and body weight classifications can be discouraged.

Body Weight of Athletes

The body weight of athletes is a function of their genetics, diet, lifestyle, training, and sport. The body weight of athletes also reflects the structural, functional, training, and performance requirements of their sport. Training efficiency of athletes also determines their body weight and composition. Brownell et al. suggest that there are three major patterns for body weight and body fatness based on the different sports. These include: 1) sports based on skill rather than physical fitness, such as golf, archery, bowling; athletes in these sports may be overweight, which can have little impact on their performance because it is mainly based on their precision and skill of execution; 2) sports with specific weight divisions for competition, such as weight lifting, wrestling, and boxing; in these sports, overall body weight is emphasized for performance as opposed to a distinction between body fat and lean mass; and 3) sports in which low body fatness is considered optimal for performance, such as running, cycling, gymnastics, diving, and figure skating; in these sports there is a strong positive association between increased performance and increased lean mass. For some of these sports, there are specific performance categories based on body weight, but there are no sport-specific body fat and lean body mass recommendations.

When discussing body weight of athletes it is important to distinguish between muscle (lean) mass and fat mass, because most athletes would benefit from greater lean mass rather than body fat mass, with a few exceptions (such as Sumo wrestlers and football players in certain positions). An athlete's body weight is defined by his or her sport, position in the sport, dietary and lifestyle practices, age, sex, and genetics. In certain weightspecific sports, such as wrestling, athletes may have certain body weight goals to meet the requirements for participation in the sport, and any body weight in excess of this goal may result in classification of the athlete as overweight, regardless of whether he is truly overweight, that is, excess body fat and BMI greater than or equal to 25. Similarly, among masters Olympic weight lifters, sex, height, and body mass are important determinants of performance; however, their relative contribution varies and is dependent on the weight class. Other groups of athletes, who are typically considered overweight because of the requirements of the sport and not necessarily due to excess body fat, include football players (certain positions), judo players, wrestlers, and weight lifters. Another group of athletes that are plagued with body weight issues are those with disabilities, and their weight issues are related both to the disability and genetic factors of these athletes. Harris et al. observed among US Special Olympic athletes, the risk of being overweight was significantly higher compared with athletes from other countries, with adult athletes from the United States being 3.1 times more likely to be overweight or obese compared with their counterparts from other countries.

Underweight

Being underweight can represent as many health concerns to an individual as being overweight can. If a person is underweight, their body may not be getting the nutrients it needs to build healthy bones, skin, and hair. While some people may have a genetic background or a medical illness that prevents them from putting on weight, there are interventions doctors can recommend to help a person gain weight.

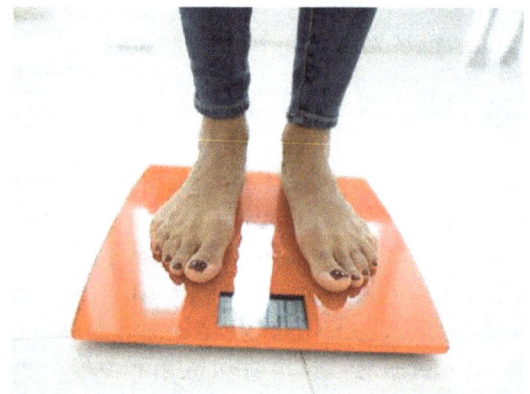

If a person's BMI is under 18.5, then they may be underweight.

The Centers for Disease Control and Prevention (CDC) recommend people use a body mass index (BMI) to calculate if they are underweight, at a healthy weight, or overweight. Using the BMI is considered a good measure of a person's weight because it compares their weight to their height. For example, a 170-pound person may not be overweight if they are very tall but could be overweight if they are very short.

Ranges for BMI include:

- Underweight: less than 18.5.

- Normal/healthy weight: 18.5 to 24.9.

- Overweight: 25.0 to 29.9.

- Obese: 30 or higher.

These calculations may be slightly inaccurate for a person who is an elite or endurance athlete whose body has a significant amount of muscle. This is because muscle weighs more than fat.

Risks of being Underweight

Being underweight can cause health problems, just as being overweight can. Not all people who are underweight experience adverse side effects or symptoms from being underweight.

However, some people, experience the following symptoms related to being underweight:

- Osteoporosis: According to a studyTrusted Source, being underweight increases a woman's risk of osteoporosis, which is where the bones are brittle and more prone to breaking.

- Skin, hair, or teeth problems: If a person does not get enough nutrients in their daily diet, they may display physical symptoms, such as thinning skin, hair loss, dry skin, or poor dental health.

- Getting sick frequently: If a person does not get enough energy from their diet to maintain a healthy body weight, they may also not be getting enough nutrients to fight off infections. As a result, a person may get sick more frequently, and common illnesses, such as a cold, can last longer than they usually would.

- Feeling tired all the time: Calories are a measurement of the energy a particular food can give a person. Not getting enough calories to maintain a healthy weight can make a person feel fatigued.

- Anemia: A person who is underweight is more likely to have low blood counts, known as anemia, which causes dizziness, headaches, and fatigue.

- Irregular periods: Women who are underweight may not have regular periods, they may find menstruation stops, or an adolescent's first period may be delayed or absent. Irregular or absent menstruation can cause infertility.

- Premature births: According to a study, a woman who is pregnant and underweight is at a higher risk for pre-term labor, which means having a baby before 37 weeks.

- Slow or impaired growth: Young people need nutrients to grow and develop healthy bones. Being underweight and not getting enough calories could mean a person may not develop as expected. Doctors call this a 'failure to thrive.'

Healthy Weight Gain Strategies

Some athletes need more calories to gain weight or maintain their weight. For example, you may need to maintain your weight for endurance sports because of the large amount of calories you burn. Endurance sports include running, swimming, and biking over long time periods or distances. Weight gain may also help to build muscle. This may help you if you participate in contact sports, such as football and hockey. A healthy weight gain goal is about ½ to 1 pound each week. Gain weight slowly to avoid gaining too much body fat. An exercise program that includes strength training will help you gain muscle weight.

Healthy Meal Plan for an Athlete

Eat a variety of healthy foods during regular meals and snacks. The following are suggested amounts of fat, carbohydrate, and protein you may need each day. Your dietitian can tell you how many calories you need each day to gain weight.

- Fat is important because it provides energy and vitamins. You need 20% to 35% of your total daily calories to come from fat. For example, a man who needs about 2900 calories per day would need 725 fat calories each day. There are both healthy fats and unhealthy fats in foods. Ask your healthcare provider for more information about different types of fat and the total amount of fat you should have.

- Carbohydrate is the main source of energy your body uses during exercise. The amount you need depends on your daily calorie needs and the sport that you do. It also depends on whether you are male or female. Athletes need 6 to 10 grams of carbohydrates for each kilogram of body weight. To find your weight in kilograms, divide your weight in pounds by 2.2. Then multiply this number by your carbohydrate needs. For example, if you weigh 70 kilograms, you would need 420 to 700 grams of carbohydrate each day.

- Protein helps to build and repair muscle, produce hormones, boost your immune system, and replace blood cells. The amount of protein you need is only slightly higher than the amount suggested for people who do not exercise. Endurance athletes need 1.2 to 1.4 grams for each kilogram of body weight per day. Athletes who do strength training (such as lifting weights) need 1.2 to 1.7 grams for each kilogram of body weight per day. People can usually meet their needs for protein by following a balanced meal plan. Good sources of protein are lean meats, poultry, eggs, milk, cheese, peanut butter, and beans. Protein or amino acid supplements are not needed for weight gain if you follow a healthy and balanced meal plan.

Increasing Calories

You need to eat or drink 500 to 1000 extra calories each day to gain about ½ to 1 pound each week. Your dietitian can tell you how many calories you need each day to gain weight. The following are some ways to add extra calories to your diet:

- Eat every 2 to 3 hours and 30 minutes after you exercise.

- Include whole-grain carbohydrates and a lean protein food in each of your meals and snacks. Examples of whole-grain carbohydrates include whole-wheat bread, rolls, and bagels. Examples of lean protein include chicken and turkey.

- Add high-calorie foods to your meals. Examples include cheese, peanut butter, avocado, nuts, and granola.

- Carry healthy snacks with you. Examples of snacks that provide about 500 calories are:

  ◦ 8 saltine crackers, 1 ounce of cheese, and 1 cup of ice cream.

  ◦ 1 cup of dry cereal with 1 cup of whole milk, 1 banana, and 1 slice of toast with 1 tablespoon of peanut butter.

  ◦ 6 graham cracker squares with 2 tablespoons of peanut butter, 2 tablespoons of raisins, and 1 cup of orange juice.

Foods with High Calorie Contents

- Choose whole-grain breads, such as honey bran, rye, and pumpernickel instead of white bread. Add peanut butter, margarine, jam, or honey for extra calories.

- Eat high-calorie cereals, such as granola and cereals that contain nuts. These are healthy choices and have more calories per serving than puffed rice or corn flakes. The serving size of a cereal is listed on the food label. You can also add more calories to cereals by adding nuts, raisins, and other fruits.

- Bananas, pineapple, mangos, raisins, dates, and dried fruit have more calories per serving than watery fruits. Some examples of watery fruits are watermelon, grapefruit, apples, and peaches. Trail mix is a good choice because it contains dried fruits and nuts.

- Add margarine, almonds, and cheese to vegetables for extra calories. Stir-frying vegetables with canola or olive oil will also add extra calories.

- Cook chicken or fish in a small amount of canola or olive oil. Red meats, such as beef, pork, and lamb, have more calories, but they also have more saturated fat. Saturated fat is an unhealthy type of fat because it may increase blood cholesterol. When you eat red meats, choose leaner cuts. Some examples of lean cuts of red meat are round or sirloin steak, ground round, fresh or boiled ham, or center loin chop.

Liquid Intake

- You can add calories to your diet by drinking juice, milk, milkshakes, and instant breakfast drinks. Drink plenty of water to prevent dehydration. Dehydration can cause serious health problems. Athletes have higher liquid needs because they lose water through sweat.

- Always carry water with you during long exercise sessions. You can wear a special bag or belt made to carry water on your back or around your waist. Drink sports drinks during exercise sessions that last longer than 1 hour. The best way to check if you are drinking enough liquids is to check the color of your urine. Urine should be clear or very light yellow, with little or no smell. If your urine is dark or smells strong, you may not be drinking enough.

Weight Gain Dietary Strategies

- Aim to include an extra 400-500 calories/day in addition to your estimated caloric requirements.

- Eat regular snacks and meals. Eat every 2-3 hours.

- Increase portion sizes at mealtimes, particularly of energy-dense foods.

- Drink juice, milk, chocolate milk or sports drinks instead of water.

- Include a smoothie or meal replacement beverage each day between meals.

- Include the use of more nutrient and energy dense foods in meal preparation such as vegetable oil, nuts and seeds, natural peanut butter, low fat dairy & dried fruit.

- Include one extra meal or two extra snacks every day.

Some other Ways to Increase Calorie Intake

- Choose hearty breads such as sprouted whole wheat (ex. Squirrelly bread), bagels, pancakes, hoagie buns, thick crusted pizza.

- Drink juices such as cranberry blends, apple, grape and pineapple instead of orange juice.

- Eat fruits such as bananas, grapes, figs, dried cranberries and apricots, persimmons, plantains.

- Use oils during cooking and sauces for accompaniments.

- Add avocado, raisins, cheese (grated or cubes), chickpeas, deli meat, olives, nuts and seeds to salads.

- Add skim milk powder or fluid milk to soups, mashed potatoes, and smoothies.

- Have toast with nut butters (peanut, almond, cashew butter) & honey or jam.

- Top baked potatoes with cottage cheese and salsa.

- Choose high calorie cereals such as granola, oatmeal and muesli and have them with milk, raisins, banana or chopped walnuts.

Calorie Boosting Snacks

- Dried fruit (fruit leather, apricots, raisins, fruit energy bars).

- Sports bars.

- Meal replacement drinks (e.g. Nutrigy, Boost, Carnation Instant Breakfast).

- Fruits (bananas, pineapple, pears).

- Granola.

- Baby carrots.

- Roasted soy nuts.

- Trail mix (nuts and dried fruit).

- Bagel with cream cheese Pudding cups.

- Low fat cereal or granola bars.

- Fig or berry newton cookies.

- Graham crackers with peanut butter.

- Sesame snaps or ginger snap cookies.

- Juice boxes (apple, cranapple, grape, pineapple, juice blends).

- Hot chocolate.

Weight Loss Strategies

Lose Fat during the Off-season

It's very difficult to decrease body fat and reach peak fitness at the same time.

To lose fat, you need to eat fewer calories. This can make training feel more difficult and prevent you from performing at your best.

For this reason, it's best to lose fat in the off-season, when you're not competing. If that's not possible, aim for less intense training periods.

Attempting fat loss in the off-season will also give you more time to reach your goal. Losing weight at a slower rate decreases the likelihood of muscle loss and seems to support better sports performance.

Most research agrees that weight loss of 1 pound (0.5 kg) or less per week is ideal.

Avoid Crash Diets

If you cut calories too drastically, your nutrient intake may not support proper training and recovery.

This can increase your risk of injury, illness, and overtraining syndrome.

The latest sports nutrition guidelines also warn against eating too few calories and reaching a dangerously low body fat percentage, both of which can disrupt reproductive function and diminish bone health.

The lowest safe recommended body fat percentage is 5% in men and 12% in women. However, these levels are not necessarily best for all athletes.

Cutting calories too quickly can also negatively affect hormones and metabolism.

To decrease body fat, athletes should eat about 300–500 fewer calories per day but avoid eating fewer than 13.5 calories per pound (30 kilocalories per kg) of fat-free mass per day.

If you don't know how much fat-free mass you have, get your body composition estimated with either a skinfold test or bioelectrical impedance analysis (BIA).

You can also get your body composition measured by dual-energy X-ray absorptiometry (DXA) or underwater weighing. These are more accurate but also tend to be expensive and harder to come by.

Eat Less Added Sugar and more Fiber

Low-carb diets providing less than 35–40% of calories from carbs seem very effective at promoting fat loss.

However, restricting carbs too dramatically is not always best for athletes. That's because it can negatively affect training and sports performance.

Aim for a carb intake that's 40% of your daily calories to maximize fat loss. Still, consume no less than 1.4–1.8 grams of carbs per pound (3–4 grams per kg) each day.

Cutting out added sugars is the healthiest way to reduce your total carb intake.

To do so, check labels and minimize foods that contain added sugars like glucose, sucrose, and fructose. Also, avoid cane juice, dextrin, maltodextrin, barley malt, caramel, fruit juice concentrate, fruit juice crystals, or other syrups.

Instead, increase your intake of vegetables high in fiber. These will help keep you fuller for longer, making you feel more satisfied.

Eat more Protein

Protein aids fat loss in several ways.

To begin with, high-protein diets increase feelings of fullness and the number of calories burned during digestion. They also help prevent muscle loss during periods of weight loss, including in well-trained athletes.

In fact, several studies show that eating 2–3 times more protein per daycan help athletes retain more muscle while losing fat.

Therefore, athletes restricting their calories to lose weight should eat 0.8–1.2 grams of protein per pound of body weight (1.8–2.7 grams per kg) per day.

That said, there's no advantage to exceeding these recommendations.

Consuming more than these amounts can displace other important nutrients, such as carbs, from your diet. This can limit your ability to train and maintain good sports performance.

Spread Protein Intake throughout the Day

In addition to eating more protein, athletes can benefit from spreading their intake throughout the day.

In fact, 20–30 grams of protein per meal seems sufficient to stimulate muscles to produce protein for the following 2–3 hours.

This is why many scientists believe that it's ideal to consume a protein-rich meal or snack every 3 hours.

Interestingly, studies in athletes show that spreading 80 grams of protein over 4 meals stimulates muscle protein production more than splitting it over 2 larger meals or 8 smaller ones.

A 2-week weight loss study in boxers also found that those who spread their daily calorie allowance over 6 meals instead of 2 lost 46% less muscle mass.

Eating a snack with 40 grams of protein immediately before bedtime can also improve recovery from training and increase muscle protein synthesis during the night.

Refuel Well after Training

Eating the right foods after training or competing is vital, especially when trying to lose body fat.

Proper refueling is especially important for days with two training sessions or when you have fewer than eight hours of recovery time between workouts and events.

Athletes following carb-restricted diets should aim to consume between 0.5–0.7 grams of carbs per pound of body weight (1–1.5 grams per kg) as soon as possible after a training session.

Adding 20–25 grams of protein can further speed up recovery and promote protein production in your muscles.

Do Strength Training

Individuals attempting to lose weight are often at risk of losing some muscle in addition to fat. Athletes are no exception.

Some muscle loss can be prevented by eating a sufficient amount of protein, avoiding crash diets, and lifting weights.

Research shows that both protein intake and strength-training exercises stimulate muscle protein synthesis. What's more, combining the two seems to produce the greatest effect.

Nevertheless, make sure to speak to your coach before adding any extra workouts to your schedule. This will reduce your risk of overtraining or injuries.

Increase Calories Gradually after you Reach your Goal

Once you've reached your body fat percentage goal, it's tempting to quickly start eating more.

However, this may not be the most effective way to maintain your results.

That's because your body can adapt to a restricted calorie intake by adjusting your metabolism and hormone levels.

Researchers believe these adaptations can persist for some time after you bump up your calorie intake and cause you to quickly regain the lost fat.

A good alternative may be to increase your calories gradually.

This may help restore your hormone levels and metabolism better, minimizing the weight regain.

Try Some of these other Weight Loss Tips

Although weight loss is a widely researched topic, the number of studies performed on athletes is limited.

Nevertheless, many of the strategies scientifically proven to help non-athletes lose body fat may also benefit athletes. Thus, you can try some of the following:

- Record your portions: Measuring your portions and keeping track of what you eat is scientifically proven to help you get better results.

- Drink enough fluids: Drinking liquids before a meal, whether it's soup or water, can help you consume up to 22% fewer calories at the meal.

- Eat slowly: Slow eaters tend to eat less and feel fuller than fast eaters. Eating slowly can help you decrease your calorie intake without feeling hungry. Aim to take at least 20 minutes for each meal.

- Avoid alcohol: Alcohol is a source of empty calories. What's more, it can prevent athletes from properly refueling after exercise, which can negatively affect future performance.

- Get enough sleep: Research suggests that too little sleep can increase hunger and appetite by up to 24%. As sleep is also important for athletic performance, make sure you get enough.

- Reduce your stress: Having high levels of stress increases cortisol levels, which promotes food cravings. Mental and physical stress can also prevent proper recovery.

Rapid Weight Loss

Rapid weight loss (RWL) has been a part of numerous sports for many decades. RWL is characterized by transitory weight loss of at least 5% of body weight in less than a week. Other than the obvious reason of dropping weight into a class where one would have advantage over lighter and weaker opponents, RWL is perceived by some as a mental toughness practice that gives them a psychological advantage over their opponents. RWL can have significant health risks for athletes. In wake of the tragic death of three collegiate wrestlers in 1997, the National Collegiate Athletic Association (NCAA) made significant changes in its rules to prevent RWL practice.

Weight-sensitive sports are among the most popular Olympic and non-Olympic sports worldwide. Most studies rely on athletes' self-report, which may not represent the true prevalence of RWL. It seems that this practice is less common among athletes in the highest weight classes of combat sports. The exact prevalence of RWL in sport is unknown. Due to many rule changes in a variety of these sports in recent years, the prevalence of RWL appears to be diminishing. Wrestling is the most commonly studied sport for RWL. Prevalence of RWL among high school, collegiate, and international style wrestlers has been reported as 40% to 90%. RWL practice is quite prevalent among other combat sports, although the accurate prevalence is unknown. RWL is also a common practice among jockeys. Multiple studies have shown that the practice of RWL starts early, often during adolescence.

Methods of RWL

The majority of athletes in weight-class sports aim to compete at the lightest weight possible in the belief that it will provide a competitive edge over their smaller and less powerful opponents. Based on sport, level of competition, weight class, age, gender, and amount of excessive weight, athletes use different active (e.g., increased exercise) and passive (e.g., low-calorie diet and heat exposure) strategies and methods to "cut" their weight rapidly. RWL is typically in the range of 5% to 10% of the athlete's body weight in a week prior to the competition. The core strategies for RWL include the following: 1) reducing food and fluid intake, 2) increasing body secretions, and 3) rising body metabolic rate to burn fat tissues. Athletes use one or several of these methods at the same time. Reducing food and fluid intake is the main strategy in RWL. Most weight-class athletes start to restrict their diet and reduce drinking fluids in the week preceding their weigh-in and gradually intensify restrictions as they get closer to the weigh-in date. In the last day before weigh-in, many athletes fast and some are so dehydrated they suck on ice cubes to prevent their mouths from excessive drying. Taking diet pills is another method for losing weight by blocking appetite and burning body fat mass. In general, athletes are interested in losing weight by maximizing fat loss while minimizing glycogen and muscle loss to benefit from lower weights while achieving a higher "strength to mass ratio" and preserving their anaerobic energy source. However, in extreme conditions, some athletes may even choose to sacrifice muscle mass by restricting protein and carbohydrate intake. Cessation of restrictive diets after weigh-in usually results in rapid weight gain due to intensified accumulation of fat mass in a mechanism known as poststarvation obesity. Repeated cycles of RWL and weight regain are associated with overall weight gain in the long term.

Reducing body weight by increasing body secretions, sweating, and dehydration is another strategy of RWL that is generally used a couple of days before weigh-in.

About 65% of the human body is made of water, which makes it a good source for significant and temporary RWL by increased sweating and dehydration. This method of cutting weight is so popular among athletes that is wellknown as "drying out". Reduced body water can be easily and rapidly regained by hydrating after weigh-in. Different methods for severe dehydration including use of wet or dry saunas, training in heated rooms, and training with plastic or rubberized suits (sweat suits) in addition to restricting fluid intake are commonly practiced by athletes in the last hours before weigh-in. It is important to note that rapid dehydration by more than 5% of the total body weight can result in serious health conditions such as muscle injuries, heat stroke, and even death and is therefore not recommended. Laxative use and intentional vomiting are other aggressive methods that are used mostly at the last day before weigh-in to minimize body weight. Although dangerous and banned by World Anti-Doping Agency, using diuretic agents is another method for RWL in the last hours before the weigh-in. Using diuretic agents is the most common anti-doping rule violation in combat sports. There are a few unusual techniques that are being used by some athletes to reduce body weight before weigh-in including enemas, chewing gum to increase salivation and then spitting out the saliva, and even shaving hairs.

Conducting strenuous exercise in the few days before weigh-in is another strategy for RWL. The overall aim of excessive exercise is to reduce body weight by utilizing body fat and even glycogen resources as well as increasing dehydration and sweating. The most common types of exercise used to achieve RWL include running, jogging, cycling, and swimming, with prolonged running or jogging at aerobic intensity in heated rooms or while wearing vaporimpermeable suits as the most common practice. Some athletes choose high-intensity intermittent exercise programs to reduce subcutaneous and abdominal body fat.

Physiological Effects

Due to the small and methodologically weak nature of existing studies, there are conflicting results on the physiological effects of RWL. It appears that RWL causes little or no increase in muscle strength and possibly can reduce it.

In a study of 17 elite male boxers, Reljic et al. did not find any alterations in the vitamin and glutathione status in the RWL group compared with those in the control group. In another study, Coswig et al. reported that mixed martial art athletes who practiced RWL (n = 5) were more likely to have abnormally high lactate dehydrogenase and aspartate aminotransferase compared with the control group (n = 12) in a regional competition in Brazil. Both groups showed increase in lactate, glucose, and cortisol levels. Degoutte et al. reported significant endocrine parameter changes (decrease in testosterone, insulin, and T3/T4 ratio and increase in adrenocorticotropic hormone (ACTH); dehydroepiandrosterone sulfate (DHEA-S) levels) in dietary restriction group (n = 10) compared with those in the control group (n = 10) after the competition.

Cognitive Function and Psychological Effects

Research on the psychological effects of RWL is not clear. A survey reported that 60% of college wrestlers and 45% of high school wrestlers felt angry while losing weight. These mood and mental performance changes could potentially impact a wrestler's school and athletic performance, although this has not been directly studied. Athletes overall are known to have more of an "iceberg" profile on their psychological scores on the validated Profile of Moods States questionnaire, with lower scores for tension, depression, and anger, high scores for vigor, and lower scores for fatigue and confusion. In the short term, athletes who cut weight can see an increase in their levels of confusion after dropping weight for competition with insignificant increases in depression and anger but another study found that decreases in weight before competition affected tension, fatigue, and anger without increasing confusion or depression. A literature review from 2012 reports decreases in memory, concentration, and self-esteem with increases in confusion, depression, rage, and fatigue after RWL. However, Choma et al. found that the effect of weight cutting on mood is not sustained after weight is regained. While Koral and Dosseville noted increases in tension and confusion with decreases in vigor after weight cutting, they posit that increases in anger and tension may result in increased performance, a theory also suggested by others.

Choma et al. also found an association between decreased mood, digit span, and story recall with hypoglycemia associated with RWL, but no changes in other cognitive tests. Other research shows no differences in cognitive testing after RWL in jockeys. It is worth mentioning that none of these studies reported improvements in psychological or cognitive parameters associated with RWL and most had control groups to offset the effect of preperformance stress on testing.

While there is concern that RWL could lead to development of eating disorders, this has not been shown. It has been reported that 10% to 15% of boys who participate in weight-sensitive sports practice unhealthy weight loss behaviors, with disordered eating the highest in weight-class sports. Surveys of in-season wrestlers have reported the use of cyclic vomiting consistent with bulimia in 1.4% to 5% of wrestlers. However, Davis et al. conducted interviews with wrestlers identified as "at risk" on the Eating Disorder Inventory Survey and concluded that the athletes' weight concerns were due entirely to the demands of wrestling and did not meet the criteria for the diagnosis of bulimia nervosa. Rouveix et al. found that athletes who participate in weight cutting are at increased risk for developing eating disorders based on predictive test scores but not on observed development of eating disorders. A large survey of judoka found no differences in weight cutting behavior between men and women and no reports of risky dieting behaviors in the off season.

Effect of RWL on Performance

Experts believe that RWL compromises sports-related aerobic and anaerobic performance. However, there is only a handful of studies in this area. In general, most studies on the effects of RWL on performance are small and have methodological weaknesses.

One of the effects of RWL is on hydration status as many RWL methods target fluid loss. Moderate dehydration (3% to 4% of body weight) impairs muscular endurance during high-intensity exercise. However, it seems that moderate dehydration does not impair maximal muscular strength or power. In a study of 28 well-trained combat athletes (wrestling, boxing, judo, taekwondo, and karate athletes), Reljic et al. reported no significant change in aerobic performance capacity in

RWL group compared with that in the control group despite a significant decrease in hemoglobin caused by impaired erythropoiesis and increased hemolysis.

Mendez et al. reported no significant changes in performance from before weight loss to after weight loss in the RWL group (n = 8) compare with the non-weight cycler group (n = 10) in a group of combat sport athletes. In another small study of 14 athletes, Artioli et al. did not find any judo-related performance deficit among experienced weight cyclers compare with that in the control group. In a study of 20 athletes, Degoutte et al. reported significant judo-related performance deficit in the RWL group compared with that in the control group. Wroble and Moxley reported in their study that high school wrestlers who practiced aggressive RWL performed better and received more medals compared with those who followed the recommended weight loss protocols. Marttinen et al. found that the self-selected RWL did not have any effect on grip strength or lower-body power among 16 male collegiate wrestlers. Studying 20 national and international judo athletes, Koral and Dosseville reported a significant decrease in judo movement repetitions over 30 s but not over 5 s in the weight loss group (n = 10) compared with that in the control group (n = 10) in France.

Wilson et al. reported significant impairment of maximum pushing frequency among eight jockeys (randomized crossover design) who rapidly lost 2% of body weight in a simulated race.

Health Consequences

Multiple medical associations and authors have warned of the potential acute and long-term medical consequences of RWL and weight cycling by athletes. Concerns about the acute health risks of weight cycling have centered primarily upon RWL of greater than 5% of body mass through extreme dehydration in the 1 to 2 days prior to weighing in. Extreme dehydration can cause decreased plasma volume, resulting in decreased stroke volume, increased heart rate, and reduced arteriovenous oxygen difference during submaximal exercise. These changes can reduce renal flow and electrolyte abnormalities and make athletes possibly more susceptible to heat injury and muscle cramps. However, these changes are quickly reversed within an hour of ad libitum fluid rehydration. The debate over the risks of RWL was indubitably altered in the fall of 1997 when three collegiate wrestlers died within a 5-wk period from complications of RWL. All three wrestlers were attempting to rapidly lose significant weight by induction of severe dehydration using traditional techniques (exercise and heat-induced sweating and fluid depravation). The practices of RWL among wrestlers could no longer be considered a harmless exercise in discipline and self-control.

Other potential health consequences of RWL and weight cycling that have been postulated include hormonal changes, growth impairment, decreased bone formation, decreased basal metabolic rate, and loss in fat-free mass with negative protein balance. However, the physiological changes observed with cyclic RWL appear to be transient and not associated with negative health consequences. Perturbations in the hypothalamic-pituitary-adrenal and growth hormone insulin-like growth factor axes were found in wrestlers during the competitive season but rapidly returned to normal after the season. Similarly, lightweight female rowers who engaged in RWL cycles were found to have decreased progesterone secretion associated with weight loss and lengthening of their menstrual cycles that returned to normal in the off season. Male and female judoist who engaged in RWL were found to have an acute net increase in bone resorption relative to formation, but this effect reversed with refeeding, and their bone mineral density was actually higher than active age-matched controls. Studies looking at the impact of weight cycling on basal metabolic rate and fat-free mass have been mixed. A longitudinal study of wrestlers found that their basal metabolic rate decreased during the wrestling season but returned to preseason values after the season and was higher than that of physically active nonwrestling controls.

There has been concern that repetitive weight loss cycling negatively affects the immune systems and reparative abilities of athletes, making them more susceptible to illness and injuries. Immune function at baseline, just prior to, and after a national championship was measured in college judoists who were classified into three groups depending on the amount of weight they lost immediately prior to the competition. Blood leukocyte, neutrophil, and lymphocyte counts were unchanged in all groups. However, the group that lost the most weight had significantly decreased phagocytic activity. Actual illness incidence was not reported for the three groups. There have been few studies looking at injury risk associated with RWL. A study done at a judo championship found that participants who lost greater than 5% of their body weight prior to the competition had a significantly greater risk of injury (36.8%) compared with athletes who did not lose weight (14.6% injury rate).

Proposed long-term consequences of frequent weight cycling include impaired growth, eating disorders, obesity, and increased cardiovascular disease risk. Two studies that monitored the growth and maturation of adolescent male wrestlers concluded that the dietary restrictions and weight cycling patterns typical of wrestlers did not adversely affect normal anthropometric growth patterns or maturation.

Large epidemiological studies have found that weight cycling in the general population is associated with an increased risk of developing type 2 diabetes mellitus and cardiovascular disease, raising concerns that athletes who engage in habitual weight cycling also could be at increased risk. Saarni et al. followed a cohort of elite Finnish athletes for 45 years. They found that former athletes from sports with weight classes gained more body mass index (BMI) units and were more likely to be obese than athletes in other sports and nonathletic controls. The enhanced weight gain was not accounted for by current health habits or baseline weight at age 20. In contrast, retired elite French athletes in weight-class sports had lower BMI and were more physically active than the age-matched general population after an average follow-up of 22 years. In addition, there was no statistical differences in weight gain between athletes who habitually weight-cycled in their careers and athletes who did not. The different findings of the studies could be at least partially due to the different periods that the athletes were active. The Finnish study looked at athletes who were active between 1920 and 1965, while the French study involved athletes active between 1978 and 2003.

Strategies to Prevent RWL Practices

The most successful way to prevent RWL methods is to implement rules that make RWL impractical. Voluntary programs that emphasized education from 1960 to 1997 did not reduce RWL. The deaths of the college wrestlers in 1997 prompted the NCAA to institute a mandatory weight monitoring program for wrestlers. The NCAA implemented five rule changes for the 1998 to 1999 season, including a minimum wrestling weight based on 5% body fat, moving weigh-ins to at most 1 h prior to competition, and a prohibition of using saunas, steam rooms, and impermeable suits to lose weight. The National Federation of State High School Associations made similar recommendations with the exception of setting the minimum at 7% body fat for boys and 12% for girls. Several studies have reported that these programs have been successful in decreasing the frequency and magnitude of RWL by wrestlers. Other weight-class sports have not implemented mandatory weight monitoring programs, although there has been a proposal for the International Judo Federation to institute a program similar to the NCAA wrestling weight certification program. At the youth level, methods of matching combat sport opponents not strictly based on weight have been successfully implemented and should be encouraged.

A study by Alderman et al. in 2004 emphasized the importance of having a rule-based weight monitoring program to effectively change athletes' behavior. The study found that high school and college wrestlers reverted to RWL methods and patterns when competing in an international tournament, which had no minimum weight rules and a longer period between the weigh-in and the competition.

Educational programs are important, in conjunction with rule changes, to change the attitude of athletes and coaches toward weight loss. RWL is ingrained in the culture of weight-class sports, particularly combat sports. For any weight management program to be successful, the athletes and coaches must believe that the medical professionals involved (physicians, athletic trainers) understand the demands of their sport. Education must focus on how healthy weight control and nutrition will make the athletes better competitors. Examples of successful wrestlers such as Kyle Dake who went up a weight class each year in college and won four NCAA championships have a greater impact on wrestlers and coaches than a discussion of possible medical risks. The American College of Sports Medicine, National Athletic Trainers Association, and International Olympic Committee Medical Commission have all published guidelines on safe weight loss and weight maintenance in athletes. These guidelines stress the importance of close working relationships between coaches, athlete trainers, physicians, and athletes to set realistic goals based on an accurate assessment of percentage of body fat. Athletes who are competing at an appropriate body composition achieved with scientifically sound training and nutrition principles will maximize their performance without needing to engage in RWL prior to the competition.

Calorie Restriction

Calorie restriction (caloric restriction or energy restriction) is a dietary regimen that reduces food intake without incurring malnutrition. "Reduce" can be defined relative to the subject's previous intake before intentionally restricting food or beverage consumption, or relative to an average person of similar body type.

Calorie restriction is typically adopted intentionally to reduce body weight. It is recommended as a possible regimen by US dietary guidelines and scientific societies for body weight control. Mild calorie restriction may be beneficial for pregnant women to reduce weight gain (without weight loss), and reduce perinatal risks for both the mother and child. For overweight or obese individuals, long-term health improvement may result from calorie restriction, although a gradual weight regain may occur.

Health Effects

Caloric intake control, and reduction for overweight individuals, is recommended by US dietary guidelines and science-based societies. Calorie restriction is recommended for people with diabetes. Mild calorie restriction may be beneficial for pregnant women to reduce weight gain (without weight loss) and reduce perinatal risks for both the mother and child. For overweight or obese individuals, calorie restriction may improve health through weight loss, although a gradual weight regain of 1–2 kg per year may occur.

Risks of Malnutrition

The term "calorie restriction" as used in the study of aging refers to dietary regimens that reduce calorie intake without incurring malnutrition. If a restricted diet is not designed to include essential nutrients, malnutrition may result in serious deleterious effects, as shown in the Minnesota Starvation Experiment. This study was conducted during World War II on a group of lean men, who restricted their calorie intake by 45% for 6 months and composed roughly 77% of their diet with carbohydrates. As expected, this malnutrition resulted in metabolic adaptations, such as decreased body fat, improved lipid profile, and decreased resting heart rate. The experiment also caused negative effects, such as anemia, edema, muscle wasting, weakness, dizziness, irritability, lethargy, and depression.

Typical low-calorie diets may not supply sufficient nutrient intake that is typically included in a calorie restriction diet.

Side Effects

People losing weight during calorie restriction risk developing side effects, such as cold sensitivity, menstrual irregularities, infertility, or hormonal changes.

Calorie Restriction For Endurance Athletes

While restricting calories may cause a reduction in weight, extreme calorie reduction has a greater impact on performance and actually creates a body composition that is often the opposite of what an athlete is trying to achieve. Over a period of time, extreme calorie reduction places the body into what is labeled "starvation mode." The primary fuel source for the brain is ketones that are derived from body fat (which is why a ketogenic diet "works"). But if the brain believes that the volume of calories being burned far exceeds the amount being consumed, then it starts to worry and a number of things happen:

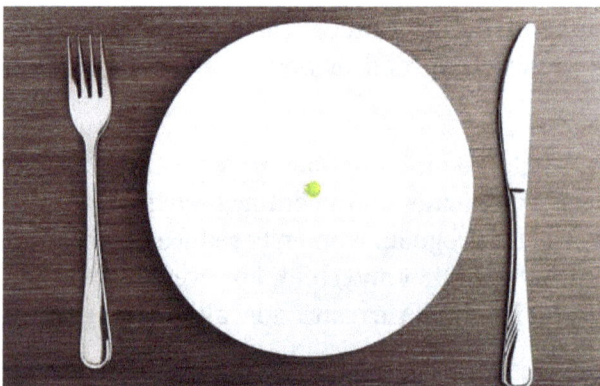

- Reduced cardiac output: Your brain will physically slow you down through the vagus nerve, which is why you may feel like you have no energy when training.

- Low glycogen stores: We can store about 1,500 calories of glycogen and this is our primary fuel source for high-intensity training. If we are not consuming enough calories to reload this, then our tank empties and we have no fuel to push our hard efforts. Ever been in a race or a hard session and you try and push harder, but your heart rate is dropping and you just cannot push? This is because the glycogen tank is empty. Glycogen takes about 24 hours to reload. If you run out during a race, it's going to be a long day.

- Reduced ability to store glycogen: In addition to not having enough glycogen to support the training session, reducing calories can also reduce the amount of glycogen the body can store effectively, reducing the size of the tank come race day.

- Muscle Breakdown I: Hard efforts cause muscle breakdown. We need energy to rebuild this muscle. No fuel means no muscle rebuild and we effectively lose strength.

- Muscle Breakdown II: If not enough energy is taken in through diet, then the body will use protein from its own muscle mass to meet its energy needs, leading to muscle wasting over time. If the individual does not consume adequate protein, then muscle will also waste as more vital cellular processes (such as respiration enzymes) recycle muscle protein for their own requirements.

- Nutrients: People who restrict calories typically restrict nutrientsessential for endurance sports such as iron, calcium, magnesium, and zinc. This is also the issue with techniques like gastric banding where the ability to consume enough nutrients is reduced.

So the effect of a large gap between calories consumed and calories expended can be summed up in two statements:

- You don't improve or you get slower.

- You maintain fat and lose muscle tone.

Meal Replacement

Meal replacements are edible products designed to allow you to skip 'sit-down' meal. Meal replacements are very popular in the world of sports nutrition. They are carefully formulated with different amounts of protein, carbohydrates and calories. Meal replacement is a huge, growing industry and to a slightly lesser extent, around the world. They can come in the form of a powder that is mixed with water or other liquids, shakes, and bars. There is a wide variety of products available at health-food stores, pharmacies, drug stores, and normal grocery stores.

Both men and women use meal replacements. When it comes to sports nutrition, different people use different types of meal replacements for entirely different goals. For example, some meal replacements help you lose weight, while others are engineered to help people put muscle or bulk up. Needless to say, it's important to choose a meal replacement wisely. While it's not a huge deal to skip a meal here or there, it's a different story if you are constantly using meal replacements as a long-term strategy. You might want to seek professional advise from either a registered sports nutritionist, sports doctor or trainer before you begin such a diet. They should be able to advise you before you embark on such an endeavor.

Using meal replacements to gain weight is a very popular technique these days with professional and amateur athletes alike. Who has time to cook properly balanced meals, right? And if you're trying to gain muscle mass, meal replacements can be a safe way to do so. Still, it's important to be very aware of what you're putting in your body. Always read the labels very carefully. Don't go overboard, and follow the recommended amounts. And of course, be careful that you don't eat or drink any meal replacements that contain foods that you are allergic to and use common sense.

Using meal replacements as a way to lose weight is an entirely different story. While meal replacements such as nutrition bars or powder shakes are relatively healthy and safe, the problem is that eating or drinking meal replacements over and over again can lead to boredom and it may be relatively easy to stray off course. Also, meal replacements often leave you wanting more because your body may be used to sitting down to a meal, chewing and swallowing a certain number of times. Even though you may be full from eating or drinking a meal replacement, you still might want to chew on something and end up eating way more than you should be.

If you do lose weight from meal replacements, it may also be difficult once you go off the diet, to keep the weight off. This is the same as with any diet. You may want to gradually reintroduce real foods into your system instead of switching from meal replacements to huge plates of food as soon as the diet is over.

Depending on the formulation, MR also possess the advantage of having a low glycemic index (GI) value; low-GI diets have been linked to improved weight maintenance and reduction in risk of diabetes and ocular disease. Many nutrition researchers and authoritative bodies around the world have highlighted the need to improve the nutrient density of diets as a means to reduce obesity while maintaining optimal nutrition status. MR also tend to be nutrient dense, meaning that they possess a high ratio of essential nutrients relative to calories.

Some markets have established clear regulatory standards and definitions for the composition and marketing claims for MR (e.g., Codex, Canada, EU, Brazil, Korea, Indonesia). However, several large markets (e.g., US, Mexico, China, Russia, India) still lack these important standards, in turn limiting research opportunities and recognition by governments, healthcare professionals and consumers of the value the category provides.

Meal Replacements for Weight Loss and Weight Maintenance

According to the most recent global analysis, obesity rates continue to rise at an alarming level overall, reaching 50% of the population in some countries, with the prevalence in women rising faster than that for men. Globally, the prevalence of obesity now exceeds that of underweight. Although obesity rates in some developed countries appear to have leveled off (e.g., US men), comorbidities, such as type II diabetes, continue to rise. The World Health Organization (WHO) estimates the prevalence of diabetes has doubled worldwide since 1980 and resulted in 3.7 million deaths in 2012, with combined direct and indirect costs estimated in the $billions annually. With overweight and obesity recognized as the strongest risk factors for type II diabetes, the WHO recommends obesity prevention, through healthy diet and physical activity, as a key approach.

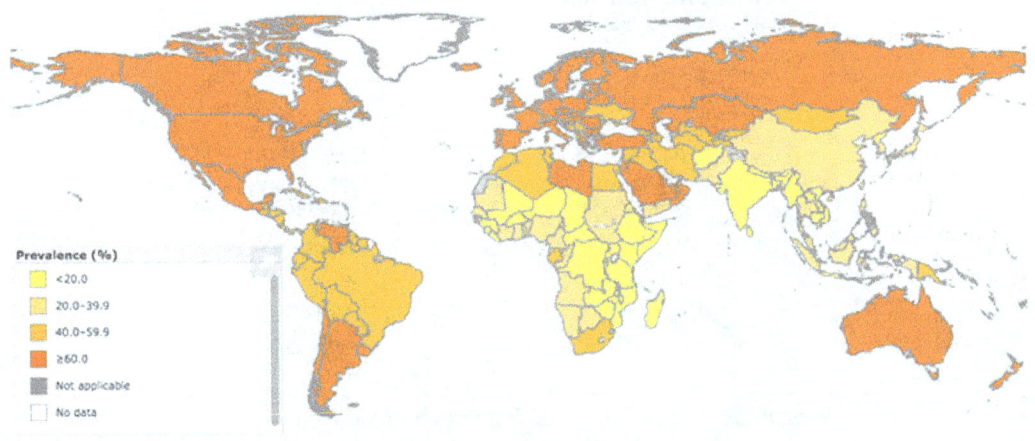

Global overweight and obesity prevalence.

Few tools have been validated as safe and effective in the treatment or prevention of obesity and overweight. Bariatric surgery is effective at treating those who are morbidly obese, yet it is associated with substantial risks and postsurgery complications, including nutrient deficiency. While advances in science and technology have eventually provided several efficacious pharmaceutical drugs for obesity treatment, the effects are modest and associated with a myriad of side effects, and many FDA-approved prescription weight loss drugs have been subsequently withdrawn from the market due to safety concerns. In contrast, nearly 150 studies demonstrate that use of MR (in various forms) safely reduces energy intake and results in sustainable weight loss. A systematic review published concluded that MR safely and effectively produce sustainable weight loss. The systematic review included six randomized, controlled MR intervention studies of at least 3 months duration, involving adults with a body mass index (BMI) ≥ 25 kg/m².

Table: Relative comparison between pharmacological, surgical and meal replacement approaches to obesity treatment and prevention.

Approach	Category	Effectiveness for obesity treatment—long term (>1 year)	Side and adverse effects
Pharmacological	Prescription drug	5% total body weight	Significant and serious, with some drugs having received FDA approval, then subsequently withdrawn from the market
Bariatric surgery	Medical device	30% of total body weight in the morbidly obese	High risks associated with surgery and postsurgery complications, including nutrient inadequacy or deficiency
Meal replacements	Conventional food and medical food	7–8% total body weight	Only nonserious (nuisance) effects reported

More recent studies have demonstrated MR effectiveness at maintaining weight loss up to several years. Intervention studies involving MR use with a year or more of follow-up have shown a range of sustained weight loss from 2% up to 11% of baseline body weight.

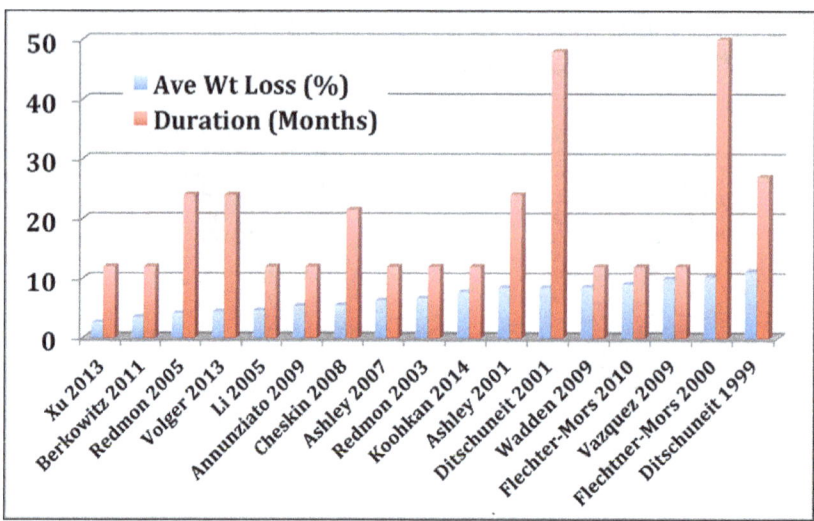

Weight loss and maintenance from randomized controlled
trials ≥1year in duration involving meal replacement.

Portion size is a key factor in determining energy intake and may be closely linked to obesity. Research indicates that portion size is directly correlated with energy intake, suggesting that controlling portion size is an effective approach to reduce energy intake and combat obesity. Among the few portion control tools researched to date, liquid MR are considered among the most effective and consistent, particularly if combined with other efforts to encourage consumption of high-nutrient-dense, low-energy-dense foods. Furthermore, MR promote adherence to a restricted calorie diet due to simple preparation and convenience compared to preparing and cooking low-calorie foods at home. MR generally contain a tight range of total calories, macro- and micronutrients, and are a nutrient-dense tool, especially useful for supporting adherence to a calorie-restricted diet through portion control.

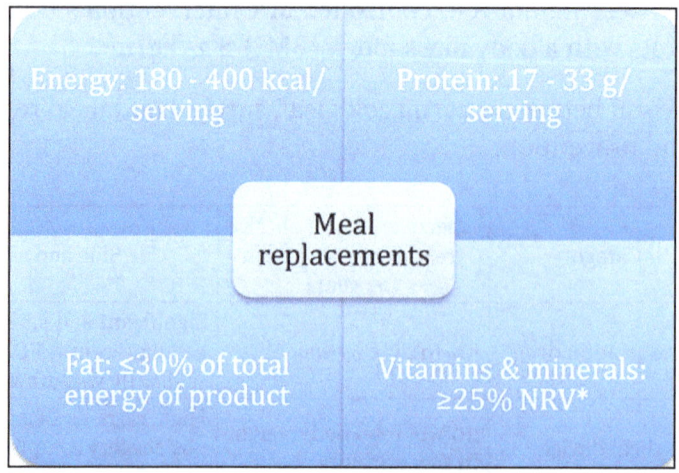

General macro- and micronutrient composition of meal replacement products.

Satiety and appetite are known to impact total energy intake, as well as food choices and eating behavior. Both are regulated by a combination of mechanical and endocrine effects ranging from the gut to the brain. With respect to diet, protein has been identified as an important contributor to satiety, defined as the absence of hunger between meals. Dietary protein can induce satiety through several mechanisms including thermic effects and induction of gut hormones such as cholecystokinin (CCK) and glucagon-like peptide 1 (GLP-1) and ghrelin. Intervention studies show that increased protein intake, using protein-enriched MR, is effective at increasing satiety, reducing hunger sensations, decreasing energy intake and facilitating weight loss in obese subjects.

Many authoritative bodies around the world have sanctioned the use of MR for weight loss and control. As far back as the mid-1980s, Codex Alimentarius recognized the use of MRs for weight control. In 2010, the European Food Safety Authority (EFSA) concluded that MR are effective for both weight loss and weight maintenance. Most recently, the Academy of Nutrition & Dietetics (AND) rated strongly the use of MR as part of a comprehensive weight management program.

Metabolic Benefits of Meal Replacement

Weight loss in obese subjects during an intervention is comprised of water, fat and lean (muscle) mass. The amount and extent of fat and muscle loss depend on the specific weight loss intervention. As lean mass determines the basal metabolic rate (BMR), the goal for any weight loss program is to lose fat mass, while preserving muscle mass. This helps to maintain a higher BMR, which in turn helps to maintain energy expenditure, which can often decline with weight loss. Use of protein-enriched MR products has been shown to effectively maintain lean body mass during weight loss, particularly when combined with resistance exercise.

Glycemic index (GI) represents a measure of the ability or rapidity of a given food to raise an individual's postprandial blood glucose level. GI is determined for a given food in reference to a standard food, usually white bread, and reflects the blood glucose-raising ability of digestible carbohydrates in a given food. Examples of relative GI values of different foods can be found in table.

Table: Glycemic index (GI) values of select foods.

High GI (≥ 70)	• Foods digested rapidly by the body and cause quick elevation in blood sugar levels
	• White bread, pretzels, and candy
Medium (56-69)	• Foods digested at a slower rate than high GI foods, causing moderate elevations in blood sugar levels
	• Apricot, oat bran, and popcorn
Low GI (≤ 55)	• Foods digested at a slower rate causing slower increases in blood sugar levels
	• Cheese, yogurt, and nuts
	• Meal replacements

A growing body of evidence suggests that the GI and glycemic load (GL, a measure of how much a given food will raise an individual's blood glucose level following consumption) of the diet play an important role in human metabolic functions and health. High GI foods and a high GL stimulate a rapid rise in insulin levels, which on a chronic basis can result in insulin resistance. The GL of a food is calculated by multiplying its GI by the amount of carbohydrate it contains per serving, and then dividing by 100. GL is a function of the amount of carbohydrate intake and the GI of the food. In contrast, GI is an inherent property of a food, independent of the amount of carbohydrate ingested. The GI value of a diet can impact insulin sensitivity and glucose metabolism. Blood sugar levels have also been implicated in appetite control, suggesting that. Furthermore, MR promote adherence to a restricted calorie diet due to simple preparation and convenience compared to preparing and cooking low-calorie foods at home. The GI of a diet may impact overall food and energy intake. Accordingly, low-GI diets have been shown to be an effective approach for managing diabetes and obesity. The combination of a high-protein, low-GI diet in obese subjects is effective at inducing weight loss and maintenance of lean body mass. Although it varies by formulation, MR tend to be high in protein and have a low GI (<55), making them ideal for incorporation into an overall low-GI diet plan.

As with insulin sensitivity, the degree of intrabdominal and visceral fat is tightly linked to metabolic syndrome. Surrounding the body's critical organs, such as the heart and liver, visceral fat stimulates systemic inflammation and is known as an increasingly serious risk factor for chronic diseases, including cardiovascular disease and diabetes. In simple terms, "sarcopenic obesity" can be defined as low skeletal muscle mass and strength combined with excess body fat, much of which is visceral fat. The concept has also been described as "thin outside, fat inside" or "TOFI". Related to obesity, individuals can have the same body mass index (BMI), but vastly different inflammatory states and risk levels due to differences in distribution and degree of visceral fat. As there is as yet no medical cure, resistance and strength exercise, combined with a high-protein diet, is recommended as one of the only effective means of addressing sarcopenic obesity and complications of excess visceral fat. When used in conjunction with reduced total calorie intake and resistance exercise, MR can also be effective at reducing visceral fat.

With respect to safety, use of MR for weight control and other metabolic benefits is among the safest approaches studied. Many individual intervention studies as well as systematic reviews have confirmed that MR safely facilitate weight loss and maintenance.

Meal Replacements and Nutritional Adequace

According to studies, individuals should consume more nutrient-dense foods to better balance meeting nutritional needs while avoiding excess calories or energy. A position paper concluded that there is a positive association between dietary energy density and increased adiposity. Nutrient density is a term referring to the amount of essential nutrients in a food relative to the amount of energy (calories) that food delivers. High-nutrient-dense foods provide a high level of nutrients with relatively low caloric value, and low-nutrient-dense foods provide a high level of calories with relatively low nutrient content. Examples of nutrient-dense foods include fruits, vegetables, whole grains, lean meats and dairy.

In the United States, more than half of the population fails to achieve the recommended intakes for key nutrients, including vitamins A, C, D and E, fiber, magnesium and potassium, all of which have been deemed "nutrients of concern" or "shortfall nutrients". Incorporation of more nutrient-dense foods into the diet is an effective approach to achieve proper nutrient adequacy without adding excess calories.

Overweight and obese individuals are at even higher risk than the general population of experiencing nutrient deficiency, particularly vitamin D. This is believed to be due, in part, to overconsumption of a high-energy-dense and low-nutrient-dense diet, a phenomenon described as "overfed but undernourished". Furthermore, weight loss regimens, particularly those involving rapid weight loss, can lead to compromised nutritional status.

With a modest amount of calories, added essential vitamins, minerals and fiber, MR are considered to be a nutrient-dense food. Indeed, a variety of studies demonstrates that use of MR during a weight control regimen helps to ensure adequate intake of essential nutrients.

References

- Malcolm Kendrick (April 12, 2015). "Why being 'overweight' means you live longer: The way scientists twist the facts". Https://www.independent.co.uk. Archived from the original on 12 April 2015. Retrieved 12 April 2015

- Sport-performance-and-body-composition, kinetic-select, education: nsca.com, Retrieved 1 June, 2019

- "BMI Classification". Global Database on Body Mass Index. World Health Organization. 2006. Archived from the original on April 18, 2009. Retrieved July 27,2012

- Weight-gain-tips-for-athletes: drugs.com, Retrieved 21 March, 2019

- 9-weight-loss-tips-for-athletes, nutrition: healthline.com, Retrieved 12 April, 2019

- US Department of Health and Human Services. (2017). "2015–2020 Dietary Guidelines for Americans - health.gov". Health.gov. Skyhorse Publishing Inc. Retrieved 30 September 2019

- Calorie-restriction-for-endurance-athletes-why-its-not-always-a-good-idea, fitness: breakingmuscle.com, Retrieved 23 June, 2019

6
Daily Meal Plans for Athletes

Different meal plans are necessary for various kinds of sports such as cricket, cycling, climbing, wrestling, bodybuilding, swimming, running, etc. This chapter sheds light on different meal plans for athletes associated with various sports to provide an in-depth understanding of the subject.

Meal Plan for a Cricketer

Cricket is a game which requires both fitness and concentration. Top level cricketers will train in cricket nets or by playing a game four or five times per week. In addition to this they will visit the gym and train with both cardiovascular equipment and weights two or three times per week. Excelling in cricket therefore takes a lot of time and energy, so it's essential to have a well structured nutrition programme to not only help you keep fit and energised for a long game, but also to help your concentration, maximising your skill potential.

Table: The meal plan is an example for an active cricketer to follow for a typical training day.

Breakfast	Large bowl of porridge made with jumbo oats + 200 ml skimmed milk + water with a tsp of sugar and raisins if desired 250 ml fresh fruit juice Tea/coffee
TRAIN	30 minutes weights moderate intensity 40 mins CV mixing high, moderate and low intensity Sip plenty of water throughout
Immediately post workout	25 g whey protein powder + 25g dextrose in water
45 minutes later	2-3 oatcakes with low fat soft cheese Item of fruit Drink
Lunch	Sandwich made with granary bread + olive oil based spread with lean ham/chicken or large mackerel fillet 100g mixed nuts & seeds Mixed salad Low fat, low sugar yoghurt Drink
Cricket training	Sip plenty of water or isotonic drink throughout
Post training	2-3 oatcakes with low fat soft cheese 100 g mixed nuts & seeds Item of fruit Drink
Evening Meal	Lean fillet steak or chicken breast or fish + herbs to taste Boiled new potatoes or basmati rice or dry roasted sweet potatoes Loads of vegetables Low fat, no added sugar yoghurt Drink
1 hour pre-bed	100 g cottage cheese/quark/low fat natural yoghurt Banana Small handful mixed nuts & seeds Drink

Porridge for breakfast is not only a hearty, filling meal, but provides slow releasing energy. Oatcakes and granary bread will top up this slow released energy through the daytime.

The diet plan provides sufficient levels of all nutrients and sustained slow released low glycaemic carbohydrates to help provide energy for long and intense training sessions.

Meal Plan for a Cyclist

Cycling is very much an endurance sport which, particularly at long distances, can place a very high demand both on the muscles and on the cardiovascular system. Typically, top cyclists will train with maybe two moderate distance sessions during the week, and one or two long distance sessions at the weekend. Roads will vary with flat and hills. In addition to the cycling training, the cyclist may visit the gym and train with weights and light machine cardiovascular work once or twice per week; the object of which is to help power, particularly in the legs. Indeed, the object of any training and diet regimen is to improve the cyclist's power to weight ratio.

Longer distance training sessions or events are very enduring and are a high demand on energy levels and will need to be followed by a couple of days rest with a high carbohydrate intake to help replenish stores.

Cyclists generally do not carry a deal of muscle mass, but will have strong leg tendon strength and excellent fitness. Following a meal plan will be ideal for a typical week's training, but both pre- and post-event carbohydrate loading is recommended in order to maximise the muscle and liver carbohydrate stores.

Breakfast	Porridge: 100 g oats + tbsp ground linseeds + 300 ml skimmed milk + tsp sugar 2 slices granary bread, toasted + olive oil based spread + natural crunchy peanut butter 250 ml fresh fruit juice Tea/coffee
Mid-morning	6 oatcakes + 200 g cottage cheese or quark Item fruit Mug green tea
Lunch	2 sandwiches made with granary bread + olive oil based spread with lean ham/chicken or large mackerel fillet 100 g mixed nuts, seeds & dried fruit Mixed salad Low fat, low sugar yoghurt Drink
Mid-afternoon	2 squares Easy Flapjacks 100g mixed nuts, seeds & dried fruit Large banana + 200 g low fat natural yoghurt Mug green tea
30 minutes pre-training	6 oatcakes Water
Running/gym training	Sip plenty of water or isotonic drink where possible

Immediately post training	20 g maltodextrin + 20 g dextrose in water
Evening meal (45 mins later)	Lean red meat or chicken breast or fish + herbs to taste Boiled new potatoes or basmati rice or dry roasted sweet potatoes or wholewheat pasta Loads of vegetables Low fat, no added sugar yoghurt Drink
Mid-evening	100 g unsweetened muesli + 250 ml skimmed milk Item fruit Drink
1 hour pre-bed	2-3 Satsuma's Small handful mixed nuts & seeds Drink

The above plan provides sufficient levels of all nutrients, however do bear in mind that the plan is merely a general guide, and there is no mention of portion sizes on purpose so that you can adapt it to suit yourself; remember men will generally require larger portions than women. You must eat a variety of different meats/fish, complex carbohydrates, fruit and vegetables every day, and drink plenty of water.

Meal Plan for a Climbers

Proper climbing nutrition starts with eating a balanced and appropriate diet with a focus on healthy nutrition. A basic climbing diet should consistent of plenty of fresh vegetables, lean proteins, whole grains, healthy fats, and unprocessed foods, plus a limited amount of refined sugar and unhealthy fats. The most important part of a solid climbing diet is to be knowledgeable about what you're putting into your body.

Pre-climb

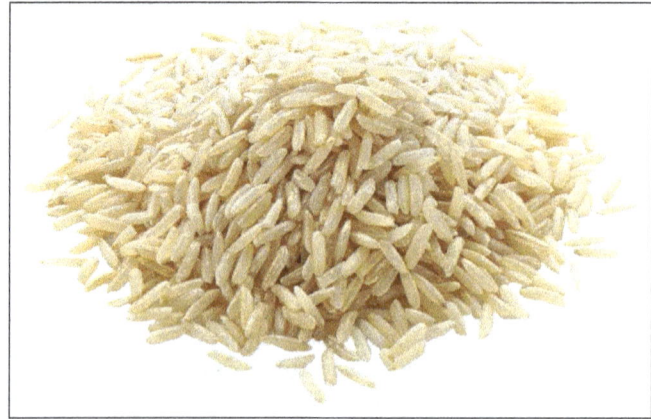

Figure out the intensity and duration of the session. You don't want to feel deprived or too full while climbing. With shorter and higher intensity climbing like bouldering, fuel up with easy-to-digest carbohydrates (dried fruit, bananas, quick oats, rice milk, or sweet potatoes). With longer and lower intensity climbing sessions like alpine climbing, include slower digesting carbohydrates (brown rice, quinoa, or beans) for sustained energy.

Consider the timing of the meal. Aim to get 25 to 30 grams of carbohydrates (a banana contains approximately 27 grams) 30 minutes before a climb. Include 20 grams of protein within 30 minutes of training or climbing to ensure that there are enough amino acids in the blood stream to prevent muscle breakdown and improve strength. Three ounces of turkey breast contains about 22 grams of protein, a ½ cup of tofu has about 20 grams, or you can get 14 grams of protein from two eggs.

Avoid fats pre-workout. They are slower to digest and could cause stomach problems while working hard.

If you eat a meal with a good balance of protein, fat, and carbohydrates one to two hours before training, you won't need to supplement with pre-workout fuel. Have a carb-protein snack 30 minutes before if it's been more than two hours since you've had a meal, or if you are putting in extra training hours. The more you train, the more nutrients you'll need to sustain energy levels.

Mid-climb

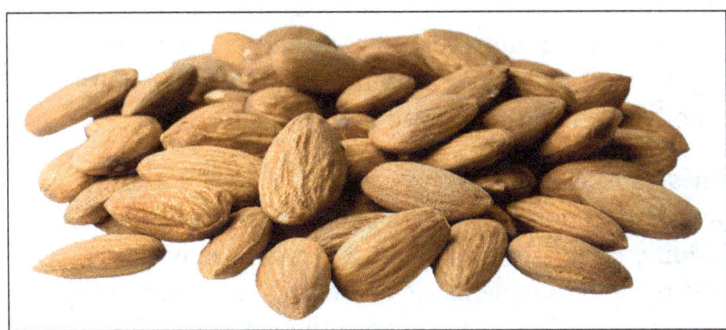

For boulderers and single-pitch sport routes, aim to replenish glycogen stores, where your body gets quick energy, every 75 to 90 minutes with 30 to 60 grams of carbs. If you have trouble keeping blood sugar stable, and going longer than an hour makes you feel irritated, fatigued, or weak, then aim to refuel every 60 minutes. Going any longer without replenishing increases the risk of muscle breakdown, fatigue, and a lower performance threshold. For short, high-intensity activities like these, high-quality carbohydrates provide excellent fuel. Choose carb sources that are slower to digest, and thus won't cause the afternoon crash. Think berries, buckwheat, wild rice, leafy greens, quinoa, sweet potatoes, yams, squash, legumes like lentils and beans, steel-cut oats, and honey or maple syrup as a sweetener. These foods are packed with vitamins, nutrients, antioxidants, and fiber, which can reduce inflammation, promote recovery, and support energy production.

For multi-pitch climbing, consume 80 to 100 grams of carbohydrates every 60 minutes. This is important for long routes that also include hard approaches. Plan to snack at belays with dehydrated fruit like mango, apricots, or apples, nut butter packets with honey or maple syrup, jerky, trail mix, and gels.

Remember to drink water every 30 minutes, especially when consuming concentrated snacks (gels).

Post-climb

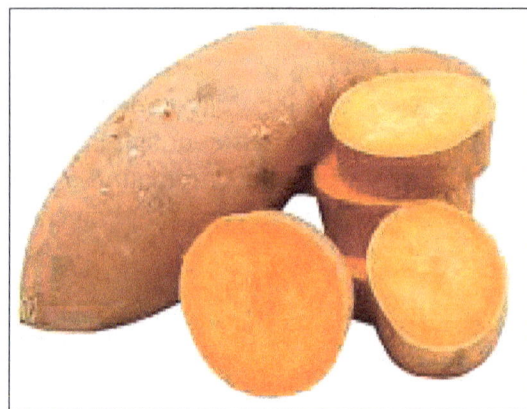

Recovery starts the minute you stop training. During prolonged activity, muscle breakdown and glycogen depletion occurs. Knowing what to eat while recovering can have a significant impact on performance. When in the recovery phase, the body replenishes glycogen stores and repairs and rebuilds muscle—if you provide the necessary nutrients.

Within 30 minutes after training, refuel with a carbohydrate and protein snack. Minimize fat intake to less than five grams; eating more than that will interfere with protein absorption and can slow digestion. Pairing 0.2 to 0.4 grams of protein per kilogram of body weight with 0.8 grams of carbs per kilogram of body weight will help you recover faster.

Stay hydrated at all times, especially in the recovery phase. This is as important as the nutrients provided. Take your body weight in pounds and cut it in half; that's how many ounces of water you should have per day, plus an additional cup for every hour of physical activity, cup of coffee, or alcoholic beverage. To make sure electrolytes are replenished as well, add an electrolyte powder to water or simply add salt to your recovery meal. Athletes can exceed the recommended daily sodium intake (1500-2400 mg) because of the large amount of fluid and salt lost through sweating. Symptoms of electrolyte deficiencies and dehydration include cramping, muscle weakness, bloating, fatigue, and headaches.

Dietary Intake

Carbohydrates

50 to 60% of daily calories, with boulderers and those increasing training hours. Sport and alpine climbers can aim for 40 to 45% of daily intake.

Protein

30 to 35% of daily calories, with sport and alpine climbers aiming to have a 10 to 15% percent more carbs than protein.

Fat

20 to 25% of daily calories for boulderers, and 25 to 35% for alpine climbers and endurance athletes aiming to have a more equal amount of fat to protein ratio and lower carbohydrate intake.

Many athletes mistakenly deprive themselves of specific foods based on the latest diet trend instead of what's best for their bodies. Cases exist where eliminating specific foods can restore health, but it can also do the opposite. Depriving the body can create nutritional deficiencies and lead to obsessive eating habits.

Carbohydrates receive a bad rap, being blamed for most digestive ailments, weight gain, and excess abdominal fat. Undoubtedly some people suffer from gluten sensitivities, but the right grains, veggies, and fruits will improve performance and promote wellness.

Optimal Weight

Achieving an optimal climbing weight can be difficult, but straightforward, healthy methods exist. Limiting refined carbs, such as white rice, white bread, baked goods and sweets, pasta, and sugar-packed snacks will help with climbing weight, performance, and health. Read nutrition labels. Most sports drinks, gels, and protein bars lack nutrients and contain excessive sugar. On long remote routes, combine real foods along with gels. Making bars from dried fruit and nuts, using honey-infused nut butter packets instead of gels, snacking on granola or jerky, and sipping coconut water or a protein shake instead of a sports drink can improve athletic function. Take the right foods to the crag instead of grabbing whatever is handy.

To maintain weight and decrease hunger, combine carbohydrate intake with protein. Consuming these two nutrients simultaneously will balance blood sugar, improve energy and mental clarity, decrease muscle breakdown, and curb sugar cravings. Hummus and veggies, berries and yogurt, tofu and brown rice, beans and rice, and chicken-topped salads all provide healthy energy and help with weight management. Divide these meals into smaller snacks to provide energy for training sessions by adjusting the serving size from a full plate to something you can grab and go.

Cutting out processed foods and refined carbohydrates, bulking up on veggies and fruit, and combining high-quality carbohydrates with protein will help with weight management.

Ketogenic Diet

Fat provides the most sustainable form of energy when trying to perform for a long time, which is why the ketogenic diet has become favored by endurance athletes. Training the body to rely on fat as the main source of fuel provides longer lasting energy without a crash, and relying on energy reserves also produces benefits like lower insulin level, improved brain health, and a decrease in chronic illness.

However, high-fat and high-protein diets are nutritionally restrictive and can cause a rebound effect—meaning your metabolism can actually slow down once you're off it. Plus, diets that emphasize extremely low carbohydrate intake can impact endocrine health. Chronic fatigue, inability to lose weight, low libido, poor recovery in between training, and change in sleep are common symptoms of adrenal fatigue as a result of dietary restriction. It's standard for someone on a ketogenic diet to consume about four grams of fat for every one gram of protein and carbohydrate. Nutrition and dietary choices should be sustainable to be successful, and this ratio is not. Simply tweaking current fat intake and exchanging foods can retrain the body and reap endurance benefits without risking the rebound effect. Reduce your refined carb intake, include nutrient- and fiber-dense carbs instead, combine healthy carbs with protein, and incorporate fats from nuts, seeds, avocados, coconut, eggs, flax, chia seeds, and even butter to help with weight management. These simple changes will improve physical and mental performance by providing key nutrients from the main food sources for recovery and sustained energy.

Healthy Digestion

Diets are only as good as the absorption. To gain the benefits of wholesome nutrition, make sure that your digestion is up to par.

Avoid foods that you are sensitive or allergic to. Common food allergens include gluten, milk, shellfish, eggs, soy, corn, citrus, some nuts, and nightshade vegetables (tomatoes, eggplant, white potatoes, bell peppers, and cayenne pepper). Although these foods are common allergens, it does not mean that everyone should avoid them—you might find that you have different allergies.

Track dietary habits and bodily reactions to discover allergic reactions. Note changes in bowel movement, mental fog or fatigue, skin issues, and increased inflammation after climbing. If you are still having negative symptoms post–food elimination, a food allergy test can uncover hidden sensitivities.

Poor digestion can also be due to a gut bacteria imbalance. Digestive tract microbiome dictate everything from mood to weight. A diet high in insoluble fiber and inulin (asparagus, artichokes, broccoli, jicama, leeks, onion, and bananas) provides plenty of prebiotics, which feed the existing bacteria. Foods high in probiotics (fermented foods like plain yogurt, kombucha, kimchi, and sauerkraut) promote a good microbiome in the gut.

Traveling can affect digestion. Most athletes complain of unintentional weight gain or changing bowel habits while traveling. To avoid this, pack plenty of "safe," non-perishable foods such as homemade bars, nuts, and dried fruit.

Meal Plan for a Wrestler

In boxing, martial arts, wrestling and MMA, fighters have to get below a target weight in order to fight in a particular weight class. Sometimes this can be a few kilos below your off-season weight, therefore there needs to be a few weeks of strict dieting to lose this excess weight, and at the same time, it's crucial to maintain muscle strength and provide adequate energy for power and hard training.

Wake	1 scoop whey protein in low sodium mineral water
8.00 am Breakfast	Porridge: 70 g oats + 200 ml skimmed milk + 2 tsp sugar 3 egg whites + 1 egg yolk scrambled
10.30 am	100g chicken breast Large banana Sip 100 ml low sodium mineral water
12.30 pm	120 g chicken breast 40 g basmati rice + tbsp sweetcorn No drink
3.00 pm	120 g chicken breast Small banana No drink

6.00 pm – weigh-in	
Immediately post weigh-in	Large Mars bar 250 ml bottle isotonic drink
Sip 1.5-2 litres of water during the next 2 hours but avoid bloating	
30 mins later	6 oatcake biscuits 1 scoop whey + 30 g dextrose in water
30 mins later	Flapjack 250 ml bottle isotonic drink
30 mins later	6 oatcakes Sweets or chocolate
Nothing apart from water 30 mins pre-fight	
After fight	Have a good meal of whatever desired to replenish

Carbohydrates need to be low in quantity, regular and of low glycaemic index (GI) choices during the daytime, like basmati rice, sweet potato and oats (porridge). Following the weigh-in carbs are a mixture of high and low GI sources. The high GI ones are to get the depleted stores up as rapidly as possible before the fight, whilst the low GI choices (oatcakes) are to stop the fighter crashing (running out of energy) in the ring, and give him/her the edge to fight longer.

Meal Plan for a Bodybuilder

The most desirable goal for most bodybuilders is to lose fat (cut) and gain muscle, but this is more complicated than it seems. from a scientific viewpoint, it isn't possible to gain muscle whilst being in an energy deficit due to the fact that muscle growth is an energy-requiring process. As you can only lose fat if you are in an energy deficit, the trick to cutting whilst gaining muscle is to fluctuate your body between energy surplus and deficit at different times of the day, or on different days of the week, through diet and exercise. Therefore on a strict cut it is not possible to gain muscle at the same time as losing body fat, as there is far too insufficient energy reserves for muscle growth, so the priority is maintaining muscle mass. But, for the main, with gentle dieting you can successfully lose fat and grow.

Following a meal plan should give a steady loss of body fat, and if you are training hard, you will keep/gain muscle. It is also reasonable in portion sizes, so should help in keeping you feeling full up and satisfied whilst cutting. This plan relies less on supplements for protein intake and more on food but still includes whey protein. There is also some flaxseed oil in there to make sure you're getting some essential fats.

Table: A sample meal plan for one day for a bodybuilder looking to lose fat whilst maintaining/gaining muscle.

Wake 7.30 am	
7.30 am	1 scoop whey protein in water
8.00am Breakfast	1-2 slices granary bread + olive oil-based spread 3 egg whites + 1 egg yolk scrambled 200 ml skimmed milk 100 ml orange juice + 1 tbsp flaxseed oil

10.30am	100-150 g chicken breast 2 oatcakes Apple
12.30pm	Tuna (100 g) + 1 tbsp low fat natural yoghurt ½ small chicken breast (60 g) 1-2 slices granary bread + olive oil based spread Huge salad
3.00pm	200 g cottage cheese/quark Banana
45 min pre-workout	80 g chicken breast 1 oatcake
TRAIN	
Immediately post workout	2 scoops whey protein in water
7.30pm	150 g white fish or 150 g lean steak/lamb/pork 2-3 boiled new potatoes or 30 g basmati rice or 40 g wholewheat pasta Vegetables/side salad
10.00pm	80 g chicken breast Stick celery/raw carrot
11.30pm	200 g cottage cheese/quark

The key to healthy quality weight gain is to eat big and eat consistently throughout the day following a structured meal plan.

Aim to eat six or seven smaller meals/snacks, rather than three big meals. Include plenty of high protein food choices, like lean meat, chicken, fish, eggs and milk; high fibre complex carbs like cereals, bread, pasta, rice and potatoes; fruit and vegetables (don't forget nuts and pulses are also good sources of protein); as well as sources of essential fats.

Timing of meals is also important - spread the meals regularly through the day, and especially important is to eat good amounts of protein and carbs after training. Some protein and weight gain supplements can also be useful aids to packing on the bulk, but not in place of good wholesome food.

Wake 7.30 am	
7.30 am	1 scoop whey protein in water
8.00 am Breakfast	Large bowl porridge made with 250 ml skimmed milk + 2 tsp sugar 2 slices granary bread toasted + olive oil-based spread Serving weight gain drink or MRP 200 ml orange juice + 1 tbsp flaxseed oil
10.30 am	2 tuna sandwiches (4 slices granary bread) Large banana
12.30 pm	Large chicken breast 200 ml fresh vegetable soup 4 slices granary bread + olive oil spread Salad Low fat yoghurt
3.00 pm	6 oatcakes Tub cottage cheese Apple
45 mins pre-workout	Glass skimmed milk Large handful mixed nuts

TRAIN	
Immediately post workout	2 scoops whey protein + 50 g dextrose in water
7.30 pm	Large bowl wholewheat breakfast cereal + 250 ml skimmed milk + 2 tsp sugar
11.30 pm	1 scoop whey protein in 150 ml skimmed milk

Meal Plan for a Swimmer

Competitive swimming varies in lengths, but it would still be seen as an endurance sport in respect of nutrition and training. However, unlike other endurance sports where power: weight ratio is of less importance, swimmers do desire a small amount of body fat surrounding the muscles to aid buoyancy; although a swimmer should be by no means 'fat', he/she may not have an exceptionally low bodyfat.

The diet should be based around low glycaemic carbohydrates for sustained energy, but with a reasonable amount of protein too, along with good amounts of essential fats, fibre, vitamins and minerals. Swimmers can be prone to muscle cramps, so, in addition to appropriate rest, ensure a good intake of electrolytes available from fruits.

Following a meal plan will be ideal for a typical swimmer to fuel training. If there's an event coming up then both pre- and post-event carbohydrate loading is recommended in order to maximise the muscle and liver carbohydrate stores.

Breakfast	Porridge: 100 g oats + tbsp ground linseeds + 300 ml skimmed milk + tsp sugar 2 slices granary bread, toasted + olive oil based spread + natural crunchy peanut butter 250 ml fresh fruit juice Tea/coffee
Mid-morning	6 oatcakes or 3-4 rye crispbread + 200 g cottage cheese or quark Handful mixed nuts Item fruit Mug green tea
Lunch	2 sandwiches made with granary bread + olive oil based spread with lean ham/chicken or large mackerel fillet or smoked salmon Tbsp sunflower seeds Mixed salad Low fat, low sugar yoghurt Drink
Mid-afternoon	2 squares Easy Flapjacks 100 g mixed nuts, seeds & dried fruit Large banana + 200 g low fat natural yoghurt Mug green tea
30 minutes pre-training	6 oatcakes 20 g whey protein powder in water Water
During training	Sip plenty of water or isotonic drink where possible

Evening meal (45 mins later)	Lean red meat or chicken/turkey breast or fish + herbs to taste Boiled new potatoes or basmati rice or dry roasted sweet potatoes or wholewheat pasta Loads of vegetables Low fat, no added sugar yoghurt Drink
Mid-Evening	100 g unsweetened muesli + 250 ml skimmed milk Item fruit Drink
1 hour pre-bed	2-3 satsumas Small handful mixed nuts & seeds Drink

Meal Plan for a Runner

Long distance running is very much endurance with a high demand on the cardiovascular system. Long distance events range from 5 km to a marathon. Training for the events will involve gym work 2-3 times per week and road running for a few kilometres 1-2 times per week, with a longer distance practice just once every few weeks. Longer distance runs are very enduring and are a high demand on energy levels. Following an event no training for a few days is essential to recuperate.

Long distance runners generally do not carry a deal of muscle mass, but will have strong leg tendon strength and excellent fitness. Following a meal plan like the one below will be ideal for a typical week's training, but both pre- and post-event carbohydrate loading is recommended in order to maximise the muscle and liver carbohydrate stores.

Breakfast	Porridge: 75 g oats + tbsp ground linseeds + 250 ml skimmed milk + tsp sugar 2 slices granary bread, toasted + olive oil based spread + natural crunchy peanut butter 250 ml fresh fruit juice Tea/coffee
Mid-morning	2-3 oatcakes + 150 g cottage cheese or quark Item fruit Mug green tea
Lunch	Sandwich made with granary bread + olive oil based spread with lean ham/chicken or large mackerel fillet 100g mixed nuts, seeds & dried fruit Mixed salad Low fat, low sugar yoghurt Drink
Mid-afternoon	2 squares Easy Flapjacks Large handful mixed nuts Large banana Mug green tea
30 minutes pre-training	2-3 oatcakes 100g mixed nuts, seeds & dried fruit Water

Running/gym training	Sip plenty of water or isotonic drink where possible
Immediately post training	20 g maltodextrin + 20 g dextrose in water
Evening meal (45 mins later)	Lean fillet steak or chicken breast or fish + herbs to taste Boiled new potatoes or basmati rice or dry roasted sweet potatoes or whole-wheat pasta Loads of vegetables Low fat, no added sugar yoghurt Drink
Mid-Evening	Unsweetened muesli + 200 ml skimmed milk Item fruit Drink
1 hour pre-bed	2-3 satsumas Small handful mixed nuts & seeds Drink

The above plan provides sufficient levels of all nutrients, however do bear in mind that the plan is merely a general guide. You must eat a variety of different meats/fish, complex carbohydrates, fruit and vegetables every day, and drink plenty of water. This plan is based around sustained slow released low glycaemic carbohydrates to help provide energy for exercise sessions. Oatcakes and granary bread will top up this slow released energy through the daytime.

References

- Cricketer, sports: mealplansite.com, Retrieved 13 May, 2019

- Cyclist, sports: mealplansite.com, Retrieved 25 February, 2019

- Nutrition-essentials-for-climbers, skills: climbing.com, Retrieved 16 January, 2019

- Fighters-making-weight, sports: mealplansite.com, Retrieved 29 March, 2019

- Bodybuilding-new-gain, sports: mealplansite.com, Retrieved 18 April, 2019

- Swimmer, sports: mealplansite.com, Retrieved 30 April, 2019

Permissions

All chapters in this book are published with permission under the Creative Commons Attribution Share Alike License or equivalent. Every chapter published in this book has been scrutinized by our experts. Their significance has been extensively debated. The topics covered herein carry significant information for a comprehensive understanding. They may even be implemented as practical applications or may be referred to as a beginning point for further studies.

We would like to thank the editorial team for lending their expertise to make the book truly unique. They have played a crucial role in the development of this book. Without their invaluable contributions this book wouldn't have been possible. They have made vital efforts to compile up to date information on the varied aspects of this subject to make this book a valuable addition to the collection of many professionals and students.

This book was conceptualized with the vision of imparting up-to-date and integrated information in this field. To ensure the same, a matchless editorial board was set up. Every individual on the board went through rigorous rounds of assessment to prove their worth. After which they invested a large part of their time researching and compiling the most relevant data for our readers.

The editorial board has been involved in producing this book since its inception. They have spent rigorous hours researching and exploring the diverse topics which have resulted in the successful publishing of this book. They have passed on their knowledge of decades through this book. To expedite this challenging task, the publisher supported the team at every step. A small team of assistant editors was also appointed to further simplify the editing procedure and attain best results for the readers.

Apart from the editorial board, the designing team has also invested a significant amount of their time in understanding the subject and creating the most relevant covers. They scrutinized every image to scout for the most suitable representation of the subject and create an appropriate cover for the book.

The publishing team has been an ardent support to the editorial, designing and production team. Their endless efforts to recruit the best for this project, has resulted in the accomplishment of this book. They are a veteran in the field of academics and their pool of knowledge is as vast as their experience in printing. Their expertise and guidance has proved useful at every step. Their uncompromising quality standards have made this book an exceptional effort. Their encouragement from time to time has been an inspiration for everyone.

The publisher and the editorial board hope that this book will prove to be a valuable piece of knowledge for students, practitioners and scholars across the globe.

Index

CPSIA information can be obtained
at www.ICGtesting.com
Printed in the USA
BVHW011026121121
621390BV00003B/59

9 781641 726979